Old-Time
Makers of Medicine

Old-Time Makers of Medicine

(Annotated)

BY

James J. Walsh

THE STORY OF THE STUDENTS AND TEACHERS OF THE SCIENCES RELATED TO MEDICINE DURING THE MIDDLE AGES

James J. Walsh, K.C.St.G., M.D.
Ph.D., LL.D., Litt.D., Sc.D.

DEAN AND PROFESSOR OF NERVOUS DISEASES AND OF THE HISTORY OF MEDICINE AT
FORDHAM UNIVERSITY SCHOOL OF MEDICINE; PROFESSOR OF PHYSIOLOGICAL
PSYCHOLOGY AT THE CATHEDRAL COLLEGE, NEW YORK

NEW YORK

1911

TO

REVEREND DANIEL J. QUINN, S.J.

The historical material here presented was gathered for my classes at Fordham University School of Medicine during your term as president of the University. It seems only fitting then, that when put into more permanent form it should appear under the patronage of your name and tell of my cordial appreciation of more than a quarter of a century of valued friendship.

"When we have thoroughly mastered contemporary science it is time to turn to past science; nothing fortifies the judgment more than this comparative study; impartiality of mind is developed thereby, the uncertainties of any system become manifest. The authority of facts is there confirmed, and we discover in the whole picture a philosophic teaching which is in itself a lesson; in other words, we learn to know, to understand, and to judge." — LITTRÉ: *Œuvres d'Hippocrate,* T. I, p. 477.

"There is not a single development, even the most advanced of contemporary medicine, which is not to be found in embryo in the medicine of the olden time." — LITTRÉ: Introduction to the Works of Hippocrates.

"How true it is that in reading this history one finds modern discoveries that are anything but discoveries, unless one supposes that they have been made twice." — DUJARDIN: *Histoire de la Chirurgie,* Paris, 1774 (quoted by Gurlt on the post title-page of his *Geschichte der Chirurgie,* Berlin, 1898)

PREFACE

The material for this book was gathered partly for lectures on the history of medicine at Fordham University School of Medicine, and partly for articles on a number of subjects in the Catholic Encyclopedia. Some of it was developed for a series of addresses at commencements of medical schools and before medical societies, on the general topic how old the new is in surgery, medicine, dentistry, and pharmacy. The information thus presented aroused so much interest, the accomplishments of the physicians and surgeons of a period that is usually thought quite sterile in medical science proved, indeed, so astonishing, that I was tempted to connect the details for a volume in the Fordham University Press series. There is no pretence to any original investigation in the history of medicine, nor to any extended consultation of original documents. I have had most of the great books that are mentioned in the course of this volume in my hands, and have given as much time to the study of them as could be afforded in the midst of a rather busy life, but I owe my information mainly to the distinguished German and French scholars who have in recent years made deep and serious studies of these Old Makers of Medicine, and I have made my acknowledgments to them in the text as opportunity presented itself.

There is just one feature of the book that may commend it to present-day readers, and that is that our medieval medical colleagues, when medicine embraced most of science, faced the problems of medicine and surgery and the allied sciences that are now interesting us, in very much the same temper of mind as we do, and very often anticipated our solutions of them—much oftener, indeed, than most of us, unless we have paid special attention to history, have any idea of. The volume does not constitute, then, a contribution to that theme that has interested the last few generations so much,—the supposed continuous progress of the race and its marvellous advance,—but rather emphasizes that puzzling question, how is it that men make important discoveries and inventions, and then, after a time, forget about them so that they have to be made over again? This is as true in medical science and in medical practice as in every other department of human effort. It does not seem possible that mankind should ever lose sight of the progress in medicine and surgery that has been made in recent years, yet the history of the past would seem to indicate that, in spite of its unlikelihood, it might well come about. Whether this is the lesson of the book or not, I shall leave readers to judge, for it was not intentionally put into it.

OUR LADY'S DAY IN HARVEST, 1911.

> "Of making many books there is no end."—
> *Eccles.* xii, 12 (circa 1000 B.C.).

> "The little by-play between Socrates and Euthydemus suggests an advanced condition of medical literature: 'Of course, you who have so many books are going in

for being a doctor,' says Socrates, and then he adds, 'there are so many books on medicine, you know.' As Dyer remarks, whatever the quality of these books may have been, their number must have been great to give point to this chaff."—*Aequanimitas,* WILLIAM OSLER, M.D., F.R.S., Blakistons, Philadelphia, 1906.

"Augescunt aliae gentes, aliae minuuntur;Inque brevi spatio mutantur saecla animantum,Et, quasi cursores vitai lampada tradunt."

—OVID.

One nation rises to supreme power in the world, while another declines, and, in a brief space of time, the sovereign people change, transmitting, like racers, the lamp of life to some other that is to succeed them.

"There is one Science of Medicine which is concerned with the inspection of health equally in all times, present, past and future." —PLATO.

I

INTRODUCTION

Under the term Old-Time Medicine most people probably think at once of Greek medicine, since that developed in what we have called ancient history, and is farthest away from us in date. As a matter of fact, however, much more is known about Greek medical writers than those of any other period except the last century or two. Our histories of medicine discuss Greek medicine at considerable length and practically all of the great makers of medicine in subsequent generations have been influenced by the Greeks. Greek physicians whose works have come down to us seem nearer to us than the medical writers of any but the last few centuries. As a consequence we know and appreciate very well as a rule how much Greek medicine accomplished, but in our admiration for the diligent observation and breadth of view of the Greeks, we are sometimes prone to think that most of the intervening generations down to comparatively recent times made very little progress and, indeed, scarcely retained what the Greeks had done. The Romans certainly justify this assumption of non-accomplishment in medicine, but then in everything intellectual Rome was never much better than a weak copy of Greek thought. In science the Romans did nothing at all worth while talking about. All their medicine they borrowed from the Greeks, adding nothing of their own. What food for thought there is in the fact, that in spite of all Rome's material greatness and wide empire, her world dominance and vaunted prosperity, we have not a single great original scientific thought from a Roman.

Though so much nearer in time medieval medicine seems much farther away from us than is Greek medicine. Most of us are quite sure that the impression of distance is due to its almost total lack of significance. It is with the idea of showing that the medieval generations, as far as was possible in their conditions, not only preserved the old Greek medicine for us in spite of the most untoward circumstances, but also tried to do whatever they could for its development, and actually did much more than is usually thought, that this story of "Old-Time Makers of Medicine" is written. It represents a period—that of the Middle Ages—that is, or was until recently, probably more misunderstood than any other in human history. The purpose of the book is to show at least the important headlands that lie along the stream of medical thought during the somewhat more than a thousand years from the fall of the Roman Empire under Augustulus (476) until the discovery of America. After that comes modern medicine, for with the sixteenth century the names and achievements of the workers in medicine are familiar—Paracelsus, Vesalius, Columbus, Servetus, Cæsalpinus, Eustachius, Varolius, Sylvius are men whose names are attached to great discoveries with which even those who are without any pretence to knowledge of medical history are not unacquainted. In spite of nearly four centuries of distance in time these men seem very close to us. Their lives will be reserved for a subsequent volume, "Our Forefathers in Medicine."

It is usually the custom to contemn the Middle Ages for their lack of interest in culture, in education, in literature, in a word, in intellectual accomplishment of any and every kind, but especially in science. There is no doubt about the occurrence of marked decadence in the intellectual life of the first half of this period. This has sometimes been attributed to what has been called the inhibitory effect of Christianity on worldly interests. Religion is said to have occupied people so much with thoughts of the other world that the beauties and wonders, as well as much of the significance, of the world around them were missed. Those who talk thus, however, forget entirely the circumstances which brought about the serious decadence of interest in culture and science at this time. The Roman Empire had been the guardian of letters and education and science. While the Romans were not original in themselves, at least they had shown intense interest in what was accomplished by the Greeks and their imitation had often risen to heights that made them worthy of consideration for themselves. They were liberal patrons of Greek art and of Greek literature, and did not neglect Greek science and Greek medicine. Galen's influence was due much more to the prominence secured by him as the result of his stay in Rome than would have been possible had he stayed in Asia. There are many other examples of Roman patronage of literature and science that might be mentioned. As we shall see, Rome drained Greece and Asia Minor of their best, and appropriated to herself the genius products of the Spanish Peninsula. Rome had a way of absorbing what was best in the provinces for herself.

Just as soon as Rome was cut off from intimate relations with the provinces by the inwandering of barbarians, intellectual decadence began. The imperial city itself had never been the source of great intellectual achievement, and the men whom we think of as important contributors to Rome's literature and philosophy were usually not born within the confines of the city. It is surprising to take a list of the names of the Latin writers whom we are accustomed to set down simply as Romans and note their birthplaces. Rome herself gave birth to but a very small percentage of them. Virgil was born at Mantua, Cicero at Arpinum, Horace out on the Sabine farm, the Plinys out of the city, Terence in Africa, Persius up in Central Italy somewhere, Livy at Padua, Martial, Quintilian, the Senecas, and Lucan in Spain. When the government of the city ceased to be such as assured opportunity for those from outside who wanted to make their way, decadence came to Roman literature. Large cities have never in history been the fruitful mothers of men who did great things. Genius, and even talent, has always been born out of the cities in which it did its work. It is easy to understand, then, the decadence of the intellectual life that took place as the Empire degenerated.

For the sake of all that it meant in the Roman Empire to look towards Rome at this time, however,it seemed better to the early Christians to establish the centre of their jurisdiction there. Necessarily, then, in all that related to the purely intellectual life, they came under the influences that were at work at Rome at this time. During the first centuries they suffered besides from the persecutions directed against them by the Emperors at various times, and these effectually prevented any external manifestations of the intellectual life on the part of Christians. It took much to overcome this serious handicap, but noteworthy progress was made in spite of obstacles, and by the time of Constantine many important officials of the Empire, the educated thinking classes of Rome, had become Christians. After the conversion of the Emperor opportunities began to be afforded, but political disturbances consequent upon barbarian influences still further weakened the old civilization until much of the intellectual life of it almost disappeared.

Gradually the barbarians, finding the Roman Empire decadent, crept in on it, and though much more of the invasion was peaceful than we have been accustomed to think, the Romans simply disappearing because family life had been destroyed, children had become infrequent, and divorce had become extremely common, it was not long before they replaced the Romans almost entirely. These new peoples had no heritage of culture, no interest in the intellectual life, no traditions of literature or science, and they had to be gradually lifted up out of their barbarism. This was the task that Christianity had to perform. That it succeeded in accomplishing it is one of the marvels of history.

The Church's first grave duty was the preservation of the old records of literature and of science. Fortunately the monasteries accomplished this task, which would have been extremely perilous for the precious treasures involved but for the favorable conditions thus afforded. Libraries up to this time were situated mainly in cities, and were subject to all the vicissitudes of fire and war and other modes of destruction that came to cities in this disturbed period. Monasteries, however, were usually situated in the country, were built very substantially and very simply, and the life in them formed the best possible safeguard against fire, which worked so much havoc in cities. As we shall see, however, not only were the old records preserved, but excerpts from them were collated and discussed and applied by means of direct observation. This led the generations to realize more and more the value of the old Greek medicine and made them take further precautions for its preservation.

The decadence of the early Middle Ages was due to the natural shifting of masses of population of this time, while the salvation of scientific and literary traditions was due to the one stable element in all these centuries—the Church. Far from Christianity inhibiting culture, it was the most important factor for its preservation, and it provided the best stimulus and incentive for its renewed development just as soon as the barbarous peoples were brought to a state of mind to appreciate it.

Bearing this in mind, it is easier to understand the course of medical traditions through the Middle Ages, and especially in the earlier period, with re gard to which our documents are comparatively scanty, and during which the disturbed conditions made medical developments impossible, and anything more than the preservation of the old authors out of the question. The torch of medical illumination lighted at the great Greek fires passes from people to people, never quenched, though often burning low because of unfavorable conditions, but sometimes with new fuel added to its flame by the contributions of genius. The early Christians took it up and kept it lighted, and, with the Jewish physicians, carried it through the troublous times of the end of the old order, and then passed it on for a while to the Arabs. Then, when favorable conditions had developed again, Christian schools and scholars gave it the opportunity to burn brightly for several centuries at the end of the Middle Ages. This medieval age is probably the most difficult period of medical history to understand properly, but it is worth while taking the trouble to follow out the thread of medical tradition from the Greeks to the Renaissance medical writers, who practically begin modern medicine for us.

It is easy to understand that Christianity's influence on medicine, instead of hampering, was most favorable. The Founder of Christianity Himself had gone about healing the sick, and care for the ailing became a prominent feature of Christian work. One of the Evangelists, St. Luke, was a physician. It was the custom a generation ago, and even later, when the Higher Criticism became popular, to impugn the tradition as to St. Luke having been a physician, but this has all been undone, and Harnack's recent book, "Luke the Physician," makes it very clear that not only the Third Gospel, but also the Acts, could only have been written by a man thoroughly familiar with the Greek medical terms of his time, and who had surely had the advantage of a training in the medical sciences at Alexandria. This makes such an important link in medical traditions that a special chapter has been devoted to it in the Appendix.

Very early in Christianity care for the ailing poor was taken up, and hospitals in our modern sense of the term became common in Christian communities. There had been military hospitals before this, and places where those who could afford to pay for service were kept during illness. Our modern city hospital, however, is a Christian institution. Besides, deformed and ailing children were cared for and homes for foundlings were established. Before Christianity the power even of life and death of the parents over their children was recognized, and deformed or ailing children, or those that for some reason were not wanted, were exposed until they died. Christianity put an end to this, and in two classes of institutions, the hospitals and the asylums, abundant opportunity for observation of illness was afforded. Just as soon as Christianity came to be free to establish its institutions publicly, hospitals became very common. The Emperor Julian, usually known as the Apostate, who hoped to re-establish the old Roman

Olympian religion, wrote to Oribasius, one of the great physicians of this time, who was also an important official of his household, that these Christians had established everywhere hospitals in which not only their own people, but also those who were not Christians, were received and cared for, and that it would be idle to hope to counteract the influence of Christianity until corresponding institutions could be erected by the government.

From the very beginning, or, at least, just as soon as reasonable freedom from persecution gave opportunity for study, Christian interest in the medical sciences began to manifest itself. Nemesius, for instance, a Bishop of Edessa in Syria, wrote toward the end of the fourth century a little work in Greek on the nature of man, which is a striking illustration of this. Nemesius was what in modern times would be called a philosopher, that is, a speculative thinker and writer, with regard to man's nature, rather than a physical scientist. He was convinced, however, that true philosophy ought to be based on a complete knowledge of man, body and soul, and that the anatomy of his body ought to be a fundamental principle. It is in this little volume that some enthusiastic students have found a description that is to them at least much more than a hint of knowledge of the circulation of the blood. Hyrtl doubts that the passage in question should be made to signify as much as has been suggested, but the occurrence of any even distant reference to such a subject at this time shows that, far from there being neglect of physical scientific questions, men were thinking seriously about them.

Just as soon as Christianity brought in a more peaceful state of affairs and had so influenced the mass of the people that its place in the intellectual life could be felt, there comes a period of cultural development represented in philosophy by the Fathers of the Church, and during which we have a series of important contributors to medical literature. The first of these was Aëtius, whose career and works are treated more fully in the chapter on "Great Physicians in Early Christian Times." He was followed by Alexander of Tralles, probably a Christian, for his brother was the architect of Santa Sophia, and by Paul of Ægina, with regard to whom we know only what is contained in his medical writings, but whose contemporaries were nearly all Christians. Their books are valuable to us, partly because they contain quotations from great Greek writers on medicine, not always otherwise available, but also because they were men who evidently knew the subject of medicine broadly and thoroughly, made observations for themselves, and controlled what they learned from the Greek forefathers in medicine by their own experience. Just at the beginning of the Middle Ages, then, under the fostering care of Christianity there is a period of considerable importance in the history of medical literature. It is one of the best proofs that we have not only that Christianity did not hamper medical development, but that, directly and indirectly, by the place that it gave to the care of the ailing in life as well as the encouragement afforded to the intellectual life, it favored medical study and writing.

A very interesting chapter in the story of the early Christian physician is to be found in what we know of the existence of women physicians in the fourth and fifth centuries. Theodosia, the mother of St. Procopius the martyr, was, according to Carptzovius, looked upon as an excellent physician in Rome in the early part of the fourth century. She suffered martyrdom under Diocletian. There was also a Nicerata who practised at Constantinople under the Emperor Arcadius. It is said that to her St. John Chrysostom owed the cure of a serious illness. From the very beginning Christian women acted as nurses, and deaconesses were put in charge of hospitals. Fabiola, at Rome, is the foundress of the first important hospital in that city. The story of these early Christian women physicians has been touched upon in the chapter on "Medieval Women Physicians," as an introduction to this interesting feature of Salernitan medical education.

During the early Christian centuries much was owed to the genius and the devotion to medicine of distinguished Jewish physicians. Their sacred and rabbinical writers always concerned themselves closely with medicine, and both the Old Testament and the Talmud must be considered as containing chapters important for the medical history of the periods in which they were written.

At all times the Jews have been distinguished for their knowledge of medicine, and all during the Middle Ages they are to be found prominent as physicians. They were among the teachers of the Arabs in the East and of the Moors in Spain. They were probably among the first professors at Salerno as well as at Montpellier. Many prominent rulers and ecclesiastics selected Jewish physicians. Some of these made distinct contributions to medicine, and a number of them deserve a place in any account of medicine in the making during the Middle Ages. One of them, Maimonides, to whom a special chapter is devoted, deserves a place among the great makers of medicine of all time, because of the influence that he exerted on his own and succeeding generations. Any story of the preservation and development of medical teaching and medical practice during the Middle Ages would be decidedly incomplete without due consideration of the work of Jewish physicians.

Western medical literature followed Roman literature in other departments, and had only the Greek traditions at second hand. During the disturbance occasioned by the invasion of the barbarians there was little opportunity for such leisure as would enable men to devote themselves with tranquillity to medical study and writing. Medical traditions were mainly preserved in the monasteries. Cassiodorus, who, after having been Imperial Prime Minister, became a monk, recommended particularly the study of medicine to the monastic brethren. With the foundation of the Benedictines, medicine became one of the favorite studies of the monks, partly for the sake of the health of the brethren themselves, and partly in order that they might be helpful to the villages that so often gathered round their monasteries. There is a well-grounded tradition that at Monte Cassino medical teaching was one of the features of the education provided there by the monks. It is generally conceded that the Benedictines had much to do with the foundation of Salerno. In the convents for women as well as the monasteries for men serious attention was given to medicine. Women studied medicine and were professors in the medical department of Salerno. Other Italian universities followed the example thus set, and so there is abundant material for the chapter on "Medieval Women Physicians."

The next phase of medical history in the medieval period brings us to the Arabs. Utterly uninterested in culture, education, or science before the time of Mohammed, with the growth of their political power and the foundation of their capitals, the Arab Caliphs took up the patronage of education. They were the rulers of the cities of Asia Minor in which Greek culture had taken so firm a hold, and captive Greece has always led its captors captive. With the leisure that came for study, Arabians took up the cultivation of the Greek philosophers, especially Aristotle, and soon turned their attention also to the Greek physicians Hippocrates and Galen. For some four hundred years then they were in the best position to carry on medical traditions. Their teachers were the Christian and Jewish physicians of the cities of Asia Minor, but soon they themselves became distinguished for their attainments, and for their medical writings. Interestingly enough, more of their distinguished men flourished in Spain than in Asia Minor. We have suggested an explanation for this in the fact that Spain had been one of the most cultured provinces of the Roman Empire, providing practically all the writers of the Silver Age of Latin literature, and evidently possessing a widely cultured people. It was into this province, not yet utterly decadent from the presence of the northern Goths, that the Moors came and readily built up a magnificent structure of culture and education on what had been the highest development of Roman civilization.

The influence of the Arabs on Western civilization, and especially on the development of science in Europe, has been much exaggerated by certain writers. Closely in touch with Greek thought and Greek literature during the eighth, ninth, and tenth centuries, it is easy to understand that the Arabian writers were far ahead of the Christian scholars of Europe of the same period, who were struggling up out of the practical chaos that had been created by the coming of the barbarians, and who, besides, had the chance for whatever Greek learning came to them only through the secondary channels of the Latin writers. Rome had been too occupied with politics and aggrandizement ever to become cultured. In spite of this heritage from the Greeks, decadence took place among the Arabs, and, as the centuries go on, what they do becomes more and more trivial, and their writing has less significance. Just the opposite happened in Europe. There, there was noteworthy progressive development until the magnificent climax of thirteenth century accomplishment was reached. It is often said that Europe owed much to the Arabs for this, but careful analysis of the factors in that progress shows that very little came from the Arabs that was good, while not a little that was unfortunate in its influence was borrowed from them with the translations of the Greek authors from that language, which constituted the main, indeed often the only, reason why Arabian writers were consulted.

With the foundation of the medical school of Salerno in the tenth century, the modern history of medical education may be said to begin, for it had many of the features that distinguish our modern university medical schools. Its professors often came from a distance and had travelled extensively for purposes of study; they attracted patients of high rank from nearly every part of Europe, and these were generous in their patronage of the school. Students came from all over, from Africa and Asia, as well as Europe, and when abuses of medical practice began to creep in, a series of laws were made creating a standard of medical education and regulating the practice of medicine, that are interesting anticipations of modern movements of the same kind. Finally a law was passed requiring three years of preliminary work in logic and philosophy before medicine might be taken up, and then four years at medicine, with a subsequent year of practice with a physician before a license to practise for one's self was issued. In addition to this there was a still more surprising feature in the handing over of the department of women's diseases to women professors, and the consequent opening up of licensure to practise medicine to a great many women in the southern part of Italy. The surprise that all this should have taken place in the south of Italy is lessened by recalling the fact that the lower end of the Italian peninsula had been early colonized by Greeks, that its name in later times was Magna Græcia, and that the stimulus of Greek tradition has always been especially favorable to the development of scientific medicine.

Salerno's influence on Bologna is not difficult to trace, and the precious tradition of surgery particularly, which was carried to the northern university, served to initiate a period of surgery lasting nearly two centuries, during which we have some of the greatest contributions to this branch of medical science that were ever made. The development of the medical school at Bologna anticipated by but a short time that of a series of schools in the north Italian universities. Padua, Piacenza, Pisa, and Vicenza had medical schools in the later Middle Ages, the works of some of whose professors have attracted attention. It was from these north Italian medical schools that the tradition of close observation in medicine and of thoroughly scientific surgery found its way to Paris. Lanfranc was the carrier of surgery, and many French students who went to Italy came back with Italian methods. In the fourteenth century Guy de Chauliac made the grand tour in Italy, and then came back to write a text-book of surgery that is one of the monuments in this department of medical science. Before his time, Montpellier had attracted attention, but now it came to be looked upon as a recognized centre of great medical teaching. The absence of the Popes from Italy and the influence of their presence at Avignon made itself felt. While culture and education declined in Italy in the midst of political disturbances, they advanced materially at the south of France.

For our generation undoubtedly the most interesting chapter in the history of medieval medicine is that which tells of the marvellous development of surgery that took place in the thirteenth and four teenth centuries. Considerable space has been devoted to this, because it represents not only an important phase of the history of medicine, and recalls the names and careers of great makers of medicine, but also because it illustrates exquisitely the possibility of important discoveries in medicine being made, applied successfully for years, and then being lost or completely forgotten, though contained in important medical books that were always available for study. The more we know of this great period in the history of surgery, the more is the surprise at how much was accomplished, and how many details of our modern surgery were anticipated. Most of us have had some inkling of the fact that anæsthesia is not new, and that at various times in the world's history men have invented methods of producing states of sensibility in which more or less painless operations were possible. Very few of us have realized, however, the perfection to which anæsthesia was developed, and the possibility this provided for the great surgeons of the later medieval centuries to do operations in all the great cavities of the body, the skull, the thorax, and the abdomen, quite as they are done in our own time and apparently with no little degree of success.

Of course, any such extensive surgical intervention even for serious affections would have been worse than useless under the septic conditions that would surely have prevailed if certain principles of antisepsis were not applied. Until comparatively recent years we have been quite confident in our assurance that antisepsis and asepsis were entirely modern developments of surgery. More knowledge, however, of the history of surgery has given a serious set-back to this self-complacency, and now we know that the later medieval surgeons understood practical antisepsis very well, and applied it successfully. They used strong wine as a dressing for their wounds, insisted on keeping them clean, and not allowing any extraneous material of any kind, ointments or the like, to be used on them. As a consequence they were able to secure excellent results in the healing of wounds, and they were inclined to boast of the fact that their incisions healed by first intention and that, indeed, the scar left after them was scarcely noticeable. We know that wine would make a good antiseptic dressing, but until we actually read the reports of the results obtained by these old surgeons, we had no idea that it could be used to such excellent purpose. Antisepsis, like anæsthesia, was marvellously anticipated by the surgical forefathers of the medieval period.

It has always seemed to me that the story of Medieval Dentistry presented an even better illustration of a great anticipatory development of surgery. This department represents only a small surgical specialty, but one which even at that period was given over to specialists, who were called dentatores. Guy de Chauliac's review of the dentistry of his time and the state of the specialty, as pictured by John of Arcoli, is likely to be particularly interesting, because if there is any department of medical practice that we are sure is comparatively recent in origin, it is dentistry. Here, however, we find that practically all our dental manipulations,the filling of teeth, artificial dentures, even orthodontia, were anticipated by the dentists of the Middle Ages. We have only the compressed account of it which is to be found in text-books of general surgery, and while in this they give mainly a heritage from the past, yet even this suffices to give us a picture very surprising in its detailed anticipation of much that we have been inclined to think of as quite modern in invention and discovery.

Medicine developed much more slowly than surgery, or, rather, lagged behind it, as it seems nearly always prone to do. Surgical problems are simple, and their solution belongs to a great extent to a handicraft. That is, after all, what chirurgy, the old form of our word surgery, means. Medical problems are more complex and involve both art and science, so that solutions of them are often merely temporary and lack finality. During the Middle Ages, however, and especially towards the end of them, the most important branches of medicine, diagnosis and therapeutics, took definite shape on the foundations that lie at the basis of our modern medical science. We hear of percussion for abdominal conditions, and of the most careful study of the pulse and the respiration. There are charts for the varying color of the urine, and of the tints of the skin. With Nicholas of Cusa there came the definite suggestion of the need of exact methods of diagnosis. A mathematician himself, he wished to introduce mathematical methods into medical diagnosis, and suggested that the pulse should be counted in connection with the water clock, the water that passed being weighed, in order to get very definite comparative values for the pulse rate under varying conditions, and also that the specific gravity of fluids from the body should be ascertained in order to get another definite datum in the knowledge of disease. It was long before these suggestions were to bear much fruit, but it is interesting to find them so clearly expressed.

At the very end of the Middle Ages came the father of modern pharmaceutical chemistry, Basil Valentine. Already the spirit that was to mean so much for scientific investigation in the Renaissance period was abroad. Valentine, however, owes little to anything except his own investigations, and they were surprisingly successful, considering the circumstances of time and place. His practical suggestions so far as drugs were concerned did not prove to have enduring value, but then this has been a fate shared by many of the masters of medicine. There were many phases of medical practice, however, that he insisted on in his works. He believed that the best agent for the cure of the disease was nature, and that the physician's main business must be to find out how nature worked, and then foster her efforts or endeavor to imitate them. He insisted, also that personal observation, both of patients and drugs, was more important than book knowledge. Indeed, he has some rather strong expressions with regard to the utter valuelessness of book information in subjects where actual experience and observation are necessary. It gives a conceit of knowledge quite unjustified by what is really known.

What is interesting about all these men is that they faced the same problems in medicine that we have to, in much the same temper of mind that we do ourselves, and that, indeed, they succeeded in solving them almost as well as we have done, in spite of all that might be looked for from the accumulation of knowledge ever since.

It was very fortunate for the after time that in the period now known as the Renaissance, after the invention of printing, there were a number of serious, unselfish scholars who devoted themselves to the publication in fine printed editions of the works of these old-time makers of medicine. If the neglect of them that characterized the eighteenth and early nineteenth centuries had been the rule at the end of the fifteenth and during the sixteenth century, we would almost surely have been without the possibility of ever knowing that so many serious physicians lived and studied and wrote large important tomes during the Middle Ages. For our forefathers of a few generations ago had very little knowledge, and almost less interest, as to the Middle Ages, which they dismissed simply as the Dark Ages, quite sure that nothing worth while could possibly have come out of the Nazareth of that time. What they knew about the people who had lived during the thousand years before 1500 only seemed to them to prove the ignorance and the depths of superstition in which they were sunk. That medieval scholars should have written books not only well worth preservation, but containing anticipations of modern knowledge, and, though of course they could not have known that, even significant advances over their own scientific conditions, would have seemed to them quite absurd.

Fortunately for us, then, the editions of the early printed books, so many of them monuments of learning and masterpieces of editorial work with regard to medieval masters of medicine, were lying in libraries waiting to be unearthed and restudied during the nineteenth century. German and French scholars, especially during the last generation, have recovered the knowledge of this thousand years of human activity, and we know now and can sympathetically study how the men of these times faced their problems, which were very much those of our own time, in almost precisely the same spirit as we do ours at the present time, and that their solutions of them are always interesting, often thorough and practical, and more frequently than we would like to think possible, resemble our own in many ways. For the possibility of this we are largely indebted originally to the scholars of the Renaissance. Without their work that of our investigators would have been quite unavailing. It is to be hoped, however, that our recovery of this period will not be followed by any further eclipse, though that seems to be almost the rule of human history, but that we shall continue to broaden our sympathetic knowledge of this wonderful medieval period, the study of which has had so many surprises in store for us.

II

GREAT PHYSICIANS IN EARLY CHRISTIAN TIMES

What we know of the life of the Founder of Christianity and how much He did for the ailing poor would make us expect that the religion that He established would foster the care and the cure of suffering humanity. As we have outlined in the Introduction, the first of the works of Christian service that was organized was the care of the sick. At first a portion of the bishop's house was given over to the shelter of the ailing, and a special order of assistants to the clergy, the deaconesses, took care of them. As Christians became more numerous, special hospitals were founded, and these became public institutions just as soon as freedom from persecution allowed the Christians the liberty to give overt expression to their feelings for the poor. While hospitals of limited capacity for such special purposes as the sheltering of slaves or of soldiers and health establishments of various kinds for the wealthy had been erected before Christianity, this was the first time that anyone who was ill, no matter what the state of his pecuniary resources, could be sure to find shelter and care. The expression of the Emperor Julian the Apostate, that admission to these hospitals was not limited to Christians, is the best possible evidence of the liberal charity that inspired them.

The ordinary passing student of the history of medicine or of hospital foundation and organization, can have no idea of the magnitude of some of these institutions, and their importance in the life of the time, unless it is especially pointed out. St. Basil, about the middle of the fourth century, erected what was spoken of as "a city for the sick," before the gates of Cæsarea. Gregory of Nazianzen, his friend, says "that well built and furnished houses stood on both sides of streets symmetrically laid out about the church, and contained rooms for the sick, and the infirm of every variety were intrusted to the care of doctors and nurses." There were separate buildings for strangers, for the poor, and for the ailing, and comfortable dwellings for the physicians and nurses. An important portion of the institution was set apart for the care of lepers, which constituted a prominent feature in Basil's work in which he himself took a special interest. Earlier in the same century Helena, the mother of the Emperor Constantine, had built similar institutions around Jerusalem, and during this same century nearly everywhere we have evidence of organization of hospitals and of care for the ailing poor.

Not only were hospitals erected, but arrangements were made for the care of the ailing poor in their own homes and for the visitation of them, and for the bringing to places adapted for their care and treatment of such as were found on the street, or neglected in their homes. The Church evidently considered itself bound to care for men's bodies as well as their souls, and many of the expressions in common use among Christians referred to this fact. Religion itself was spoken of as a medicine of the soul and the body. Christianity was defined as the religion of healing. The word salvation had a reference to both body and soul. Baptism was spoken of as the bath of the soul, the holy Eucharist as the elixir of immortal life, and penance as the medicine of the soul. It is not surprising to find, then, that Harnack has found among the texts that illustrate the history of early Christian literature this one: "In every community there shall be at least one widow appointed to assist women who are stricken with illness, and this widow shall be trained in her duties, neat and careful in her ways, shall not be self-seeking, must not indulge too freely in wine in order that she may be able to take up her duties at night as well as by day, and shall consider it her duty to keep the Church officials informed of all that seems necessary."

The saving of deformed and ailing infants or children whose parents did not care to have the trouble of rearing them, required the establishment by the Christians of another set of institutions, Foundling Asylums and Hospitals for Children. Until the coming of Christianity parents were supposed to have the right of life and death over their children, and no one questioned it. In every country in the world until the coming of Christianity this had always been the case. Besides, there were institutions for the care of the old. These are the classes of mankind who are especially liable to suffer from disease, and the opportunity to study human ailments in such institutions could scarcely help but provide facilities for clinical observation such as had not existed before. Unfortunately the work of Christianity was hampered, first by the Roman persecutions, and then later by the invasion of the barbarians, who had to be educated and lifted up to a higher plane of civilization before they could be brought to appreciate the value of medical science, much less contribute to its development.

Harnack, whose writings in the higher criticism of Scripture have attracted so much attention in recent years, began his career in the study of Christian antiquities with a monograph on Medical Features of Early Christianity. [1] He mentions altogether some sixteen physicians who reached distinction in the earliest days of Christianity. Some of these were priests, some of them bishops, as Theodotos of Laodicea; Eusebius, Bishop of Rome; Basilios, Bishop of Ancyra, and at least one, Hierakas, was the founder of a religious order. The first Christian physicians came mainly from Syria, as might be expected, for here the old Greek medical traditions were active. Among them must be enumerated Cosmas and Damian, physicians who were martyred in the persecution of Diocletian, and who have been chosen as the patrons of the medical profession. Justinian erected a famous church to them. It became the scene of pilgrimages. Organizations of various kinds since, as the College of St.Come, and medical societies, have been named after them.

Some idea of the interest of ecclesiastics in medical affairs may be gathered from a letter of Bishop Theodoret of Cyrus, directed to the prefect of the city, when he was about to leave the place. He wrote (see Puschmann, Vol. I., p. 494): "When I took up the Bishopric of Cyrus I made every effort to bring in from all sides the arts that would be useful to the people. I succeeded in persuading skilled physicians to take up their residence here. Among these is a very pious priest, Peter, who practises medicine with great skill, and is well known for his care for the people. Now that I am about to leave the city, some of those who came at my invitation are preparing also to go. Peter seems resolved to do this. I appeal to your highness, therefore, in order to commend him to your special care. He handles patients with great skill and brings about many cures."

Distinguished Christian writers and scholars, and the Fathers of the Church in the early centuries, evidently paid much attention to medicine. Tertullian speaks of medical science as the sister of philosophy, and has many references to the medical doctrines discussed in his time. Lactantius, in his work, "De Opificio Dei," has much to say with regard to the human body as representing the necessity for design in creation. His teleological arguments have much more force now than they would have had for people generally twenty years ago. We have come back to recognize the place of teleology. Clement of Alexandria was an early Christian temperance advocate, who argued that the use of wine was only justified when it did good as a medicine. The problems of embryology and of diseases of childhood interested him as they did many other of the early Christian writers.

AËTIUS

The first great Christian physician whose works meant much for his own time, and whose writings have become a classic in medicine, was Aëtius Amidenus, that is, Aëtius of Amida, who was born in the town of that name in Mesopotamia, on the upper Tigris (now Diarbekir), and who flourished about the middle of the sixth century. His medical studies, as he has told us himself, were made at Alexandria. After having attracted attention by his medical learning and skill, he became physician to one of the emperors at Byzantium, very probably Justinian, (527-565). He seems to have been succeeded in the special post that was created for him at court by Alexander of Tralles, the second of the great Christian physicians. There is no doubt that Aëtius was a Christian, for he mentions Christian mysteries, and appeals to the name of the Saviour and the martyrs. He was evidently a man of wide reading, for he quotes from practically every important medical writer before his time. Indeed, he is most valuable for the history of medicine, because he gives us some idea of the mode of treatment of various subjects by predecessors whose fame we know, but none of whose works have come to us. His official career and the patronage of the Emperor, the breadth of his scholarship, and the thoroughly practical character of his teaching, show how medical science and medical art were being developed and encouraged at this time.

Aëtius' work that is preserved for us is known in medical literature as his sixteen books on medical practice. In most of the manuscript it is divided into four Tetrabibloi, or four book parts, each of which consists of four sections called Logoi in Greek, Sermones in Latin. This work embraces all the departments of medicine, and has a considerable portion devoted to surgery, but most of the important operations and the chapters on fractures and dislocations are lacking. Aëtius himself announces that he had prepared a special work on surgery, but this is lost. Doubtless the important chapters that we have noted as lacking in his work would be found in this. He is much richer in pathology than most of the older writers, at least of the Christian era; for instance, Gurlt says that he treats this feature of the subject much more extensively even than Paulus Æginetus, but most of his work is devoted to therapeutics.

At times those who read these old books from certain modern standpoints are surprised to find such noteworthy differences between writers on medicine, who are separated sometimes only by a generation, and sometimes by not more than a century, in what regards the comparative amount of space given to pathology, etiology, and therapeutics. Just exactly the same differences exist in our own day, however. We all know that for those who want pathology and etiology the work of one of our great teachers is to be consulted, while for therapeutics it is better to go to someone else. When we find such differences among the men of the olden time we are not so apt to look at them with sympathetic discrimination, as we do with regard to our contemporaries. We may even set them down to ignorance rather than specialization of interest. These differences depend on the attitude of mind of the physician, and are largely the result of his own personal equation. They do not reflect in any way either on his judgment or on the special knowledge of his time, but are the index of his special receptivity and teaching habit.

Aëtius' first and second books are taken up entirely with drugs. The first book contains a list of drugs arranged according to the Greek alphabet. In the third book other remedial measures, dietetic, manipulative, and even operative, are suggested. In these are included venesection, the opening of an artery, cupping, leeches, and the like. The fourth and fifth books take up hygiene, special dietetics, and general pathology. In the sixth book what the Germans call special pathology and therapy begins with the diseases of the head. The first chapter treats of hydrocephalus. In this same book rabies is treated. What Aëtius has consists mainly of quotations from previous authors, many of whom he had evidently read with great care.

Concerning those "bitten by a rabid dog or those who fear water," Gurlt has quoted the following expression, with regard to which most people will be quite ready to agree with him when he says that it contains a great deal of truth, usually thought to be of much later origin: "When, therefore, any one has been bitten by a rabid dog the treatment of the wound must be undertaken just as soon as possible, even though the bite should be small and only superficial. One thing is certain, that none of those who are not rightly treated escape the fatal effect. The first thing to do is to make the wound larger, the mouth of it being divided and dilated by the scalpel. Then every portion of it and the surrounding tissues must be firmly pressed upon with the definite purpose of causing a large efflux of blood from the part. Then the wound should be deeply cauterized, etc."

There are special chapters devoted to eye and ear diseases, and to various affections of the face. Under this the question of tattooing and its removal comes in. It is surprising how much Aëtius has with regard to such nasal affections as polyps and ulcers and bleedings from the nose. In this book, however, he treats only of their medicinal treatment. What he has to say about affections of the teeth is so interesting that it deserves a paragraph or two by itself.

He had much to say with regard to the nervous supply of the mucous membranes of the gums, tongue, and mouth, and taught that the teeth received nerves through the small hole existing at the end of every root. For children cutting teeth he advised the chewing of hard objects, and thought that the chewing of rather hard materials was good also for the teeth of adults. For fistulas leading to the roots of teeth he suggests various irritant treatments, and, if they do not succeed, recommends the removal of the teeth. He seems to have known much about affections of the gums and recognizes a benignant and malignant epulis. He thought that one form of epulis was due to inflammation of a chronic character, and suggests that if remedies do not succeed it should be removed. His work is of interest mainly as showing that even at this time, when the desire for information of this kind is usually supposed to have been in abeyance, physicians were gathering information about all sorts even of the minor ailments of mankind, gathering what had been written about them, commenting on it, adding their own observations, and in general trying to solve the problems as well as they could.

Aëtius seems to have had a pretty good idea of diphtheria. He speaks of it in connection with other throat manifestations under the heading of "crusty and pestilent ulcers of the tonsils." He divides the anginas generally into four kinds. The first consists of inflammation of the fauces with the classic symptoms, the second presents no inflammation of the mouth nor of the fauces, but is complicated by a sense of suffocation—apparently our croup. The third consists of external and internal inflammation of the mouth and throat, extending towards the chin. The fourth is an affection rather of the neck, due to an inflammation of the vertebræ—retropharyngeal abscess—that may be followed by luxation and is complicated by great difficulty of respiration. All of these have as a common symptom difficulty of swallowing. This is greater in one variety than in another at different times. In certain affections even "drinks when taken are returned through the nose."

Hypertrophy of the tonsils—Aëtius speaks of them as glands—is to be treated by various astringent remedies, but if these fail the structures should be excised. His description of the excision is rather clear and detailed. The patient should be put in a good full light, and the mouth should be held open and each gland pulled forward by a hook and excised. The operator should be careful, however, only to excise those portions that are beyond the natural size, for if any of the natural substance of the gland is cut into, or if the incision is made beyond the projecting portion of the tonsil, there is grave danger of serious hemorrhage. After excision a mixture of water and vinegar should be kept in the mouth for some time. This should be administered cold in order to prevent the flow of blood. After this very cold water should be taken.

In this same book, Chapter L, he treats of foreign bodies in the respiratory and upper digestive tracts. If there is anything in the larynx or the bronchial tubes the attempt must be made to secure its ejection by the production of coughing or sneezing. If the foreign body can be seen it should be grasped with a pincers and removed. If it is in the esophagus, Aëtius suggests that the patient should be made to swallow a sponge dipped in grease, or a piece of fat meat, to either of which a string has been attached, in order that the foreign body may be caught and drawn out. If it seems preferable to carry the body on into the stomach, the swallowing of large mouthfuls of fresh bread or other such material is recommended.

With regard to goitre, Aëtius has some interesting details. He says that "all tumors occurring in the throat region are called bronchoceles, for every tumor among the ancients was called a cele, and, though the name is common to them, they differ very much from one another." Some of them are fatty, some of them are pultaceous, some of them are cancerous, and some of them he calls honey tumors, because of a honey-like humor they contain. "Sometimes they are due to a local dilatation of the blood vessels, and this is most frequently connected with parturition, apparently being due to the drawing of the breath being prevented or repressed during the most violent pains of the patient. Such local dilatation at this point of the veins is incurable, but there are also hard tumors like scirrhus and malignant tumors, and those of great size. With the exception of these last, *all the tumors of this region are easily cured,* yielding either to surgery or to remedies. Surgery must be adapted to the special tumor, whether it be honey-like or fatty, or pultaceous." The prognosis of goitrous tumors is much better than might be expected, but evidently Aëtius saw a number of the functional disturbances and enlargements of the thyroid gland, which are so variable in character as apparently to be quite amenable to treatment.

Aëtius' treatment of the subject of varicosities is quite complete in its suggestions. "The term varices," he says, "is applied to dilated veins, which occur sometimes in connection with the testes and sometimes in the limbs. Operations on testicular varices patients do not readily consent to; those on the limbs may be cured in several ways.First, simple section of the skin lying above the dilated vessel is made, and with the hook it is separated from the neighboring tissues and tied. After this the dilated portion is removed and pressure applied by means of a bandage. The patient is ordered to remain quiet, but with the legs higher than the head. Some people prefer treatment by means of the cautery." Gurlt, in his "History of Surgery," calls attention to the fact that two of our modern methods of treating varicose veins are thus discussed in Aëtius, that by ligation and that by the cautery. The cautery was applied over a space the breadth of a finger at several points along the dilated veins.

Aëtius' chapters on obstetrics and gynæcology are of special interest, because, while we are prone to think that gynæcology particularly is a comparatively modern development of surgery, this surgical authority of the early Middle Ages treats it rather exhaustively. His sixteenth book is for the most part (one hundred and eleven chapters of it) devoted to these two subjects. He has a number of interesting details in the first thirty-six chapters with regard to conception, pregnancy, labor, and lactation, which show how practical were the views of the physicians of the time. Gurlt has given us some details of his chapters on diseases of the breast. Aëtius differentiates phagedenic and rodent ulcers and cancer. All the ordinary forms of phagedenic ulcer yield to treatment, while malignant growths are rendered worse by them. Where ulcers are old, he suggests the removal of their thickened edges by the cautery, for this hastens cure and prevents hemorrhage. With regard to cancer, he quotes from Archigenes and Leonides. He says that these tumors are very frequent in women, and quite rare in men. Even at this time cancer had been observed and recognized in the male breast. He emphasizes the fact that cancerous nodules become prominent and become attached to surrounding tissues. There are two forms, those with ulcer, and those without. He describes the enlargement of the veins that follows, the actual varicosities, and the dusky or livid redness of the parts which seem to be soft, but are really very hard. He says that they are often complicated by very painful conditions, and that they cause enlargement of the glands and of the arms. The pain may spread to the clavicle and the scapula, and he seems to think that it is the pain that causes the enlargement of the glands at a distance.

His description of ulcerative cancer of the breast is very striking. He says that it erodes without cause, penetrating ever deeper and deeper, and cannot be stopped until it emits a secretion worse than the poison of wild beasts, copious and abominable to the smell. With these other symptoms pains are present. This form of cancer is especially made worse by drugs and by all manner of manipulation. The paragraph from Leonides quoted by Aëtius gives a description of operation for cancer of the breast, in which he insists particularly on the extensive removal of tissue and the free use of the cautery. "The cautery is used at first in order to prevent bleeding, but also because it helps to destroy the remains of diseased tissues. When the burning is deep, prognosis is much better. Even in cases where indurated tumors of the breast occur that might be removed without danger of bleeding, it is better to use the cautery freely, though the amputation of such a portion down to the healthy parts may suffice." Aëtius quotes this with approval.

Others before Aëtius had suggested the connection between hypertrophy of the clitoris and certain exaggerated manifestations of the sexual instinct, and the development of vicious sexual habits. As might be expected from this first great Christian physician and surgeon, he emphasizes this etiology for certain cases, and outlines an operation for it. This operation had been suggested before, but Aëtius goes into it in detail and describes just how the operation should be done, so as to secure complete amputation of the enlarged organ, yet without injury. He warns of the danger of removing more than just the structure itself, because this may give rise to ugly and bothersome scars. After the operation a sponge wet with astringent wine should be applied, or cold water, especially if there is much tendency to bleeding, and afterwards a sponge with manna or frankincense scattered over it should be bound on. He treats of other pathological conditions of the female genitalia, varicose veins, growths of various kinds, hypertrophy of the *portio vaginalis uteri*, an operation for which is described, and of various tumors. He describes epithelioma very clearly, enumerates its most frequent locations in their order, lays down its bad prognosis, and hence the necessity for early operation with entire removal of the new growth whenever possible. He feared hemorrhage very much, however, and warns with regard to it, and evidently had had some very unfortunate experiences in the treatment of these conditions.

Aëtius seems to have had as thoroughly scientific an interest in certain phases of chemistry apart from medicine as any educated physician of the modern time might have. Mr. A. P. Laurie, in his "Materials of the Printer's Craft,"[2] calls attention to the fact that the earliest reference to the use of drying oil for varnish is made by the physician Aëtius.

Aëtius, or Aëtios, to use for the nonce the Greek spelling of his name, which sometimes occurs in medical literature, and should be known, has been the subject of very varied estimation at different times. About the time of the Renaissance he was one of the first of the early writers on medicine accorded the honor of printing, and then was reprinted many times, so that his estimation was very high. With the reawakening of clinical medicine in the seventeenth century his reputation waxed again, and Boerhaave declared that the works of Aëtius had as much importance for physicians as had the Pandects of Justinian for lawyers. This high estimation had survived almost from the time of the Renaissance, when Cornelius went so far as to say: "Believe me, that whoever is deeply desirous of studying things medical, if he would have the whole of Galen abbreviated and the whole of Oribasius extended, and the whole of Paulus (of Ægina) amplified, if he would have all the special remedies of the old physicians as well in pharmacy as in surgery boiled down to a summa for all affections, he will find it in Aëtius." Naturally enough, this exaggerated estimation was followed by a reaction, in which Aëtius came to be valued at much less than he deserved. After all is taken into account in the vicissitudes of his fame, it is clear, however, that he is one of the most important links in the chain of medical tradition, and himself worthy to be classed among makers of medicine for his personal observations and efforts to pass on the teachings of the old to succeeding generations.

ALEXANDER OF TRALLES

An even more striking example than the life and work of Aëtius as evidence for the encouragement and patronage of medicine in early Christian times, is to be found in the career of Alexander of Tralles, whose writings have been the subject of most careful attention in the Renaissance period and in our own, and who must be considered one of the great independent thinkers in medicine. While it is usually assumed that whatever there was of medical writing during the Middle Ages was mere copying and compilation, here at least is a man who could not only judiciously select, but who could critically estimate the value of medical opinions and procedure, and weighing them by his own experience and observation, turn out work that was valuable for all succeeding generations. The modern German school of medical historians have agreed in declaring him an independent thinker and physician,who represents a distinct link in medical tradition.

He came of a distinguished family, in which the following of medicine as a profession might be looked upon as hereditary. His father was a physician, and it is probable that there were physicians in preceding generations, and one of his brothers, Dioscoros, was also a successful physician. Altogether four of his brothers reached such distinction in their life work that their names have come down to us through nearly fifteen hundred years. The eldest of them was Anthemios, the builder of the great church of Santa Sophia in Constantinople. As this is one of the world's great churches, and still stands for the admiration of men a millennium and a half after its completion, it is easy to understand that Anthemios' reputation is well founded. A second brother was Metrodoros, a distinguished grammarian and teacher, especially of the youthful nobility of Byzantium, as it was then called, or Constantinople, as we have come to call it. A third brother was a prominent jurist, also in Constantinople. The fourth brother, Dioscoros, like Alexander, a physician, remained in his birthplace, Tralles, and acquired there a great practice.

It was with his father at Tralles that Alexander received his early medical training. The father of a friend and colleague, Cosmas, who later dedicated a book to Alexander, was also his teacher, while he was in his native city. As a young man, Alexander undertook extensive travels, which led him into Italy, Gaul, Spain, and Africa, everywhere gathering medical knowledge and medical experience. Then he settled down at Rome, probably in an official position, and practised medicine successfully until a very old age. He was probably eighty years of age when, some time during the first decade of the seventh century, he died.

Puschmann, who has made a special study of Alexander's life and work, suggests that since some of his books have the form of academic lectures he was probably a teacher of medicine at Rome. As might be expected from what we know of the relations of the rest of the family to the nobility of the time, it is easy to understand, especially in connection with hints in Alexander's favorite modes of therapeutics, that costliness of remedies made no difference to his patients, that he must have had the treatment of some of the wealthiest families in Rome.

His principal work is a Treatise on the Pathology and Therapeutics of Internal Diseases, in twelve books. The first eleven books were evidently material gathered for lectures or teaching of some kind. The twelfth book, in which considerable use of Aëtius' writings is made, was written, according to Puschmann, toward the end of Alexander's life, and was meant to contain supplementary matter, comprising especially his views gathered from observation as to the pathology of internal diseases. A shorter treatise of Alexander is with regard to intestinal parasites. There are many printed editions of these books, and many manuscript copies are in existence. Alexander was often quoted during the Middle Ages, and in recent years, with the growth of our knowledge of medical history, he has come to be a favorite subject of study.

Alexander's first book of pathology and therapeutics treats of head and brain diseases. For baldness, the first symptom of which is falling out of the hair, he counsels cutting the hair short, washing the scalp vigorously, and the rubbing in of sulphur ointments. For grey hair he suggests certain hair dyes, as nutgalls, red wine, and so forth. For dandruff, which he described as the excessive formation of small flake-like scales, he recommends rubbing with wine, with certain salves, and washing with salt water.

He gives a good deal of attention to diseases of the nervous system. He has a rather interesting chapter on headache. The affection occurs in connection with fevers, after excess in drinking, and as a consequence of injury to the skull. Besides, it develops as a result of disturbances of the natural processes in the head, the stomach, the liver, and the spleen. Headache, as the first symptom of inflammation of the brain, is often the forerunner of convulsions, delirium, and sudden death. Chronic or recurrent headache occurs in connection with plethora, diseases of the brain, biliousness, digestive disturbances, insomnia, and continued worry. Hemicrania has its origin in the brain, because of the presence of toxic materials, and specially their transformation into gaseous substances. It also occurs in connection with abdominal affections. This latter remark particularly is directed to the cases which occur in women.

For apoplexy and the consequent paralysis, Alexander considered venesection the best remedy. Massage, rubbings, baths, and warm applications are recommended for the paralytic conditions. He had evidently had considerable experience with epilepsy. It develops either from injuries of the head or from disturbances of the stomach, or occasionally other parts of the body. When it occurs in nursing infants, nourishment is the best remedy, and he gives detailed directions for the selection of a wet nurse, and very careful directions as to her mode of life. He emphasizes very much the necessity for careful attention to the gastro-intestinal tract in many cases of epilepsy. Planned diet and regular bowels are very helpful. He rejects treatment of the condition by surgery of the head, either by trephining or by incisions, or cauterization. Regular exercise, baths, sexual abstinence are the foundation of any successful treatment. It is probable that we have returned to Alexander's treatment of epilepsy much more nearly than is generally thought. There are those who still think that remedies of various kinds do good, but in the large epileptic colonies regular exercise, bland diet, regulation of the bowels, and avoidance of excesses of all kinds, with occupation of mind, constitute the mainstay of their treatment.

Alexander has much to say with regard to phrenitis, a febrile condition complicated by delirium, which, following Galen, he considers an affection of the brain. It is evidently the brain fever of the generations preceding the last, an important element of which was made up of the infectious meningitises. Alexander suggests its treatment by opiates after preliminary venesection, rubbings, lukewarm baths, and stimulating drinks. Every disturbance of the patient must be avoided, and visitors must be forbidden. The patient's room should rather be light than dark. His teaching crops up constantly in the centuries after his time, until the end of the nineteenth century, and while we now understand the causes of the condition better, we can do little more for it than he did.

Alexander divided mental diseases into two, the maniacal and melancholic. Mania was, however, really a further development of melancholia, and represented a high grade of insanity. Under melancholy he groups not only what we denominate by that term, but also all depressed conditions, and the paranoias, as also many cases of imbecility. The cause of mental diseases was to be found in the blood. He counselled the use of venesection, of laxatives and purgatives, of baths and stimulant remedies. He insisted very much, however, on mental influence in the disease, on change of place and air, visits to the theatre, and every possible form of mental diversion, as among the best remedial measures.

After his book on diseases of the head, his most important section is on diseases of the respiratory system. In this he treats first of angina, and recommends as gargles at the beginning light astringents; later stronger astringents, as alum and soda dissolved in warm water, should be employed. Warm compresses, venesection from the sublingual veins, and from the jugular, and purgatives in severe cases, are the further remedies. He treats of cough as a symptom due to hot or cold, dry or wet dyscrasias. Opium preparations carefully used are the best remedies. The breathing in of steam impregnated with various ethereal resins, was also recommended.

He gives a rather interestingly modern treatment of consumption. He recommends an abundance of milk with a strong nutritious diet, as digestible as possible. A good auxiliary to this treatment was change of air, a sea voyage, and a stay at a watering-place. Asses' and mares' milk are much better for these patients than cows' and goats' milk. There is not enough difference in the composition of these various milks to make their special consumption of import, but it is probable that the suggestive influence of the taking of an unusual milk had a very favorable effect upon patients, and this effect was renewed frequently, so that much good was ultimately accomplished. For hemoptysis, especially when it was acute and due as Alexander thought to the rupture of a blood vessel in the lungs, he recommended the opening of a vein at the elbow or the ankle—in order to divert the blood from the place of rupture to the healthy parts of the circulation. He insisted that the patients must rest, that they should take acid and astringent drinks, that cold compresses should be placed upon the chest (our ice bags), and that they should take only a liquid diet at most lukewarm, or, better, if agreeable to them, cold. When the bleeding stopped, a milk cure was very useful for the restoration of these patients to strength.

It is not surprising, then, to find that Alexander suggests a thoroughly rational treatment for pleurisy. He recognizes this as an inflammation of the membrane covering the ribs, and its symptoms are severe pain, disturbance of breathing, and coughing. In certain cases there is severe fever, and Alexander knows of purulent pleurisy, and the fact that when pus is present the side on which it is is warmer than the other. Pleurisy can be, he says, rather easily confounded with certain liver affections, but there is a peculiar hardness of the pulse characteristic of pleurisy, and there is no expectoration in liver cases, though it also may be absent in many cases of pleurisy. Sufferers from liver disease usually have a paler color than pleuritics. His treatment consists in venesection, purgatives, and, when pus is formed, local incision. He recommends the laying on of sponges dipped in warm water, and the internal use of honey lemonade. Opium should not be used unless the patient suffers from sleeplessness.

Some of the general principles of therapeutics that Alexander lays down are very interesting, even from our modern standpoint. Trust should not be placed in any single method of treatment. Every available means of bringing relief to the patient should be tried. "The duty of the physician is to cool what is hot, to warm what is cold, to dry what is moist, and to moisten what is dry. He should look upon the patient as a besieged city, and try to rescue him with every means that art and science places at his command. The physician should be an inventor, and think out new ways and means by which the cure of the patient's affection and the relief of his symptoms may be brought about." The most important factor in his therapeutics is diet.Watering-places and various forms of mineral waters, as well as warm baths and sea baths, are constantly recommended by him. He took strong ground against the use of many drugs, and the rage for operating. The prophylaxis of disease is in Alexander's opinion the important part of the physician's duty. His treatment of fever shows the application of his principle: cold baths, cold compresses, and a cooling diet, were his favorite remedies. He encouraged diaphoresis nearly always, and gave wine and stimulating drugs only when the patient was very weak. He differentiates two kinds of quartan fever. One of these he attributes to an affection of the spleen, because he had noticed that the spleen was enlarged during it, and that, after purgation, the enlarged spleen decreased in size.

Alexander was a strong opponent of drastic remedies of all kinds. He did not believe in strong purgatives, nor in profuse and sudden blood-lettings. He opposed arteriotomy for this reason, and refused to employ extensive cauterization. His diagnosis is thorough and careful. He insisted particularly on inspection and palpation of the whole body; on careful examination of the urine, of the feces, and the sputum; on study of the pulse and the breathing. He thought that a great deal might be learned from the patient's history. The general constitution is also of importance. His therapeutics is, above all, individual. Remedies must be administered with careful reference to the constitution, the age, the sex, and the condition of the patient's strength. Special attention must always be paid to nature's efforts to cure, and these must be en couraged as far as possible. Alexander had no sympathy at all with the idea that remedies must work against nature. His position in this matter places him among the dozen men whose name and writings have given them an enduring place in the favor of the profession at all times, when we were not being carried away by some therapeutic fad or imagining that some new theory solved the whole problem of the causation and cure of disease.

Gurlt, in his "History of Surgery," has abstracted from Alexander particularly certain phases of what the Germans call external pathology and therapeutics. For instance, Alexander's treatment of troubles connected with the ear is very interesting. Gurlt declares that this chapter alone provides striking evidence for Alexander's practical experience and power of observation, as well as for his knowledge of the literature of medicine. He considers that only a short abstract is needed to show that.

For water that has found its way into the external ear, Alexander suggests a mode of treatment that is still popularly used. The patient should stand upon the leg corresponding to the side on which there is water in his ear, and then, with head leaning to that side, should hop or kick out with the other leg. The water may be drawn out by means of suction through a reed. In order to get foreign bodies out of the external auditory canal, an ear spoon or other small instrument should be wrapped in wool and dipped in turpentine, or some other sticky material. Occasionally he has seen sneezing, especially if the mouth and nose are covered with a cloth, and the head leant toward the affected side, bring about a dislodgment of the foreign body. If these means do not succeed, gentle injections of warm oil or washing out of the canal with honey water should be tried. Foreign bodies may also be removed by means of suction. Insects or worms that find their way into the ear may be killed by injections of acid and oil, or other substances.

Gurlt also calls attention to Alexander's careful differentiation of certain very dangerous forms of inflammation of the throat from others which are rather readily treated. He says, "Inflammation of the throat may, under certain circumstances, belong to the severest diseases. The patients succumb to it as a consequence of suffocation, just as if they were choked or hanged. For this reason, perhaps, the affection bears the name synanche, which means constriction." He then points out various other forms of inflammation of the throat, acute and chronic, suggesting various names and the differential diagnostic signs.

One of the most surprising chapters of Alexander's knowledge of pathology and therapeutics is to be found in his treatment of the subject of intestinal worms, which is contained in a letter sent by him to his friend, Theodore, whose child was suffering from them. He describes the *oxyuris vermicularis* with knowledge manifestly derived from personal observation. He dwells on the itching in the region of the anus, caused by the *oxyuris,* and the fact that they probably find their way into the upper part of the digestive tract because of the soiling of the hands. He knew that the tapeworms often reached great length,—he has seen one over sixteen feet long,—and also that they had a life cycle, so that they existed in two different forms. He describes the roundworms as existing in the intestines, but occasionally wandering into the stomach to be vomited. His vermifuges were the flowers and the seeds of the pomegranate, the seeds of the heliotrope, castor-oil, and certain herbs that are still used, by country people, at least, as worm medicines. For roundworms he recommended especially a decoction of *artemisia maritima,* coriander seeds, and decoctions of thyme. Our return to thymol for intestinal parasites is interesting. For the *oxyuris* he prescribed clysters of ethereal oils. We have not advanced much in our treatment of intestinal worms in the fifteen hundred years since Alexander's time.

PAUL OF ÆGINA

Another extremely important writer in these early medieval times, whose opportunities for study in medicine and for the practice of it, were afforded him by Christian schools and Christian hospitals, was Paul of Ægina. He was born on the island of Ægina, hence the name Æginetus, by which he is commonly known. There used to be considerable doubt as to just when Paul lived, and dates for his career were placed as widely apart as the fifth and the seventh centuries. We know that he was educated at the University of Alexandria. As that institution was broken up at the time of the capture of the city by the Arabs, he cannot have been there later than during the first half of the seventh century. An Arabian writer, Abul Farag, in "The Story of the Reign of the Emperor Heraclius," who died 641, says that "among the celebrated physicians who flourished at this time was Paulus Æginetus." In his works Paul quotes from Alexander of Tralles, so that there seems to be no doubt now that his life must be placed in the seventh century.

The most important portion of Paul's work for the modern time is contained in his sixth book on surgery. In this his personal observations are especially accumulated. Gurlt has reviewed it at considerable length, devoting altogether nearly thirty pages to it, and it well deserves this lengthy abstract. Paul quotes a great many of the writers on surgery before his time, and then adds the results of his own observation and experience. In it one finds careful detailed descriptions of many operations that are usually supposed to be modern. Very probably the description quoted by Gurlt of the method of treating fishbones that have become caught in the throat will give the best idea of how thoroughly practical Paul is in his directions. He says: "It will often happen in eating that fishbones or other objects may be swallowed and get caught in some part of the throat. If they can be seen they should be removed with the forceps designed for that purpose. Where they are deeper, some recommend that the patient should swallow large mouthfuls of bread or other such food. Others recommend that a clean soft sponge of small circumference to which a string is attached be swallowed,and then drawn out by means of the string. This should be repeated until the bone or other object gets caught in the sponge and is drawn out. If the patient is seen immediately after eating, and the swallowed object is not visible, vomiting should be brought on by means of a finger in the throat or irritation with the feather, and then not infrequently the swallowed object will be brought up with the vomit."

In the chapter immediately following this, XXXIII, there is a description of the method of opening the larynx or the trachea, with the indications for this operation. The surgeon will know that he has opened the trachea when the air streams out of the wound with some force, and the voice is lost. As soon as the danger of suffocation is over, the edges of the wound should be freshened and the skin surfaces brought together with sutures. Only the skin without the cartilage should be sutured, and general treatment for encouraging union should be employed. If the wound fails to heal immediately, a treatment calculated to encourage granulations should be undertaken. This same method of treatment will be of service whenever we happen to have a patient who, in order to commit suicide, has cut his throat. Paul's exact term is, perhaps, best translated by the expression, slashed his larynx.

One of the features of Paul's "Treatise on Surgery" is his description of a radical operation for hernia. He describes scrotal hernia under the name enterocele, and says that it is due either to a tearing or a stretching of the peritoneum. It may be the consequence either of injury or of violent efforts made during crying. When the scrotum contains only omentum, he calls the condition epiplocele; when it also contains intestine, an epiplo-enterocele. Hernia that does not descend into the scrotum he calls bubonocele. For operation the patient should be placed on the back, and, the skin of the inguinal region being stretched by an assistant, an oblique incision in the direction in which the blood vessels run should be made. The incision should then be stretched by means of retractors, until the contents of the sac can be lifted out. All adhesions should be broken up and the fat be removed, and the hernia replaced within the abdomen. Care should be taken that no loop of intestine is allowed to remain. Then a large needle with double thread made of ten strands should be run through the middle of the incision in the end of the peritoneum, and tied firmly in cross sutures. The outer structures should be brought together with a second ligature, and the lower end of the incision should have a wick placed in it for drainage, and the site of operation should be covered with an oil bandage.

The Arab writer, Abul Farag, to whose references we owe the definite placing of the time when Paul lived, said that "he had special experience in women's diseases, and had devoted himself to them with great industry and success. The midwives of the time were accustomed to go to him and ask his counsel with regard to accidents that happen during and after parturition. He willingly imparted his information, and told them what they should do. For this reason he came to be known as the Obstetrician." Perhaps the term should be translated the man-midwife, for it was rather unusual for men to have much knowledge of this subject. His knowledge of the phenomena of menstruation was as wide and definite. He knew a great deal of how to treat its disturbances. He seems to have been the first one to suggest that in metrorrhagia, with severe hemorrhage from the uterus, the bleeding might be stopped by putting ligatures around the limbs. This same method has been suggested for severe hemorrhage from the lungs as well as from the uterus in our own time. In hysteria he also suggested ligature of the limbs, and it is easy to understand that this might be a very strongly suggestive treatment for the severer forms of hysteria. It is possible, too, that the modification of the circulation to the nervous system induced by the shutting off of the circulation in large areas of the body might very well have a favorable physical effect in this affection. Paul's description of the use of the speculum is as complete as that in any modern text-book of gynæcology.

FURTHER CHRISTIAN PHYSICIANS

Another distinguished Christian medical scientist was Theophilus Protosbatharius, who belonged to the court of the Greek Emperor Heraclius, in the seventh century. He seems to have had a life very full of interest and surprisingly varied duties. He was a bishop, and, at the same time, commander of the imperial bodyguard, and the author of a little work on the fabric of the human body. The most surprising chapter in the history of the book is that for some two centuries, in quite modern times, it was used as a text-book of anatomy at the University of Paris. It was printed in a number of editions early in the history of printing, at least one very probably before 1500, and several later.

There are very interesting phases of medicine delightfully surprising in their modernity to be found here and there in many of these early Christian writers on medicine. For instance, in a compend of medicine written by one Leo, who, under the Emperor Theophilus, seems to have been a prominent physician of Byzantium (the compend was written for a young physician just beginning practice), we find the following classification of hydrops or abdominal dilatation: "There are three kinds; the first is ascites, due to the presence of watery fluid, for which we do paracentesis; second, tympany, when the abdomen is swollen from the presence of air or gas. This may be differentiated by percussion of the belly. When air is present the sound given forth is like that of a drum, while in the first form ascites the sound is like that from a sack [the word used is the same as for a wine sack]; the third form is called anasarca, when the whole body swells."

It has often been the subject of misunderstanding as to why medicine should have developed among the Latin Christian nations so much more slowly than among the Arabs during the early Middle Ages. Anyone who knows the conditions in which Christianity came into existence in Italy will not be surprised at that. The Arabs in the East were in contact with Greek thought, and that is eminently prolific and inspiring. At the most, the Christians in Italy got their inspiration at second hand through the Romans. The Romans themselves, in spite of intimate contact with Greek physicians, never made any important contributions to medical science, nor to science of any kind. Their successors, the Christians of Rome and Italy, then could scarcely be expected to do better, hampered especially, as they were, by the trying social conditions created by the invasion of the barbarians from the North. Whenever the Christians were in contact with Greek thought and Greek medicine, above all, as at Alexandria, or in certain of the cities of the near East, we have distinguished contributions from them.

ARABIAN CHRISTIAN PHYSICIANS

That this is not a partial view suggested by the desire to make out a better case for Christianity in its relation to science will be very well understood, besides, from the fact that a number of the original physicians of Arab stock who attracted attention during the first period of Arabian medicine, that is, during the eighth and ninth centuries, were Christians. There are a series of physicians belonging to the Christian family Bachtischua, a name which is derived from Bocht Jesu, that is, servant of Jesus, who, from the middle of the eighth to the middle of the eleventh century, acquired great fame. The first of them, George (Dschordschis), after acquiring fame elsewhere, was called to Bagdad by the Caliph El-Mansur, where, because of his medical skill, he reached the highest honors. His son became the body-physician of Harun al-Raschid.In the third generation Gabriel (Dschibril) acquired fame and did much, as had his father and grandfather, for the medicine of the time, by translations of the Greek physicians into Arabian.

These men may well be said to have introduced Greek medicine to the Mohammedans. It was their teaching that aroused Moslem scholars from the apathy that had characterized the attitude of the Arabian people toward science at the beginning of Mohammedanism. As time went on, other great Christian medical teachers distinguished themselves among the Arabs. Of these the most prominent was Messui the elder, who is also known as Janus Damascenus. Both he and his father practised medicine with great success in Bagdad, and his son became the body-physician to Harun al-Raschid either after or in conjunction with Gabriel Bachtischua. Like his colleague or predecessor in official position, he, too, made translations from the Greek into Arabic. Another distinguished Arabian Christian physician was Serapion the elder. He was born in Damascus, and flourished about the middle of the ninth century. He wrote a book on medicine called the "Aggregator," or "Breviarium," or "Practica Medicinæ," which appeared in many printed editions within the century after the invention of printing. During the ninth century, also, we have an account of Honein Ben Ischak, who is known in the West as Johannitius. After travelling much, especially in Greece and Persia, he settled in Bagdad, and, under the patronage of the Caliph Mamum, made many translations. He translated most of the old Greek medical writers, and also certain of the Greek philosophic and mathematical works. The accuracy of his translations became a proverb. His compendium of Galen was the text-book of medicine in the West for many centuries. It was known as the "Isagoge in Artem Parvam Galeni." His son, Ishac Ben Honein, and his nephew, Hobeisch, were also famous as medical practitioners and translators.

Still another of these Arabian Christians, who acquired a reputation as writers in medicine, was Alkindus. He wrote with regard to nearly everything, however, and so came to be called the philosopher. He is said altogether to have written and translated about two hundred works, of which twenty-two treat of medicine. He was a contemporary of Honein Ben Ischak in the ninth century. Another of the great ninth-century Christian physicians and translators from the Greek was Kostaben Luka. He was of Greek origin, but lived in Armenia and made translations from Greek into Arabic. Nearly all of these men took not alone medical science, but the whole round of physical science, for their special subject. A typical example in the ninth century was Abuhassan Ben Korra, many of whose family during succeeding generations attracted attention as scholars. He became the astronomer and physician of the Caliph Motadhid. His translations in medical literature were mainly excerpts from Hippocrates and Galen meant for popular use. These Christian translators, thoroughly scientific as far as their times permitted them to be, were wonderfully industrious in their work as translators, great teachers in every sense of the word, and they are the men who formed the traditions on which the greater Arabian physicians from Rhazes onward were educated.

It would be easy to think that these men, occupied so much with translations, and intent on the re-introduction of Greek medicine, might have depended very little on their own observations, and been very impractical. All that is needed to counteract any such false impression, however, is to know something definite about their books. Gurlt, in his "History of Surgery," has some quotations from Serapion the elder, who is often quoted by Rhazes. In the treatment of hemorrhoids Serapion advises ligature and insists that they must be tied with a silk thread or with some other strong thread, and then relief will come. He says some people burn them *medicinis acutis* (touching with acids, as some do even yet), and some incise them with a knife. He prefers the ligature, however. He calmly discusses the removal of stones from the kidney by incision of the pelvis of the kidney through an opening in the loin. He considers the operation very dangerous, however, but seems to think the removal of a stone from the bladder a rather simple procedure. His description of the technique of the use of a catheter and of a stylet with it, and apparently also of a guide for it in difficult cases, is extremely interesting. He suggests the opening of the bladder in the median line, midway between the scrotum and the anus, and the placing of a canula therein, so as to permit drainage until healing occurs.

Even this brief review of the careers and the writings of the physicians of early Christian times shows how well the tradition of old Greek medicine was being carried on. There was much to hamper the cultivation of science in the disturbances of the time, the gradual breaking up of the Roman Empire, and the replacement of the peoples of southern Europe by the northern nations, who had come in, yet in spite of all this, medical tradition was well preserved. The most prominent of the conservators were themselves men whose opinions on problems of practical medicine were often of value, and whose powers of observation frequently cannot but be admired. There is absolutely no trace of anything like opposition to the development of medical science or medical practice, but, on the contrary, everywhere among political and ecclesiastical authorities, we find encouragement and patronage. The very fact that, in the storm and stress of the succeeding centuries, manuscript copies of the writings of the physicians of this time were preserved for us in spite of the many vicissitudes to which they were subjected from fire, and war, and accidents of various kinds for hundreds of years, until the coming of printing, shows in what estimation they were held. During this time they owed their preservation to churchmen, for the libraries and the copying-rooms were all under ecclesiastical control.

III

GREAT JEWISH PHYSICIANS[3]

Any account of Old-Time Makers of Medicine without a chapter on the Jewish Physicians would indeed be incomplete. They are among the most important factors in medieval medicine, representing one of the most significant elements of medical progress. In spite of the disadvantages under which their race labored because of the popular feeling against them on the part of the Christians in the earlier centuries and of the Mohammedans later, men of genius from the race succeeded in making their influence felt not only on their own times, but accomplished so much in making and writing medicine as to influence many subsequent generations. Living the segregated life that as a rule they had to, from the earliest times (the Ghettos have only disappeared in the nineteenth century), it would seem almost impossible for them to have done great intellectual work. It is one of the very common illusions, however, that great intellectual work is accomplished mainly in the midst of comfortable circumstances and as the result of encouraging conditions. Most of our great makers of medicine at all times, and never more so than during the past century, have been the sons of the poor, who have had to earn their own living, as a rule, before they reached manhood, and who have always had the spur of that necessity which has been so well called the mother of invention. Their hard living conditions probably rather favored than hampered their intellectual accomplishments.

It is not unlikely that the difficult personal circumstances in which the Jews were placed had a good deal to do at all times with stimulating their ambitions and making them accomplish all that was in them. Certain it is that at all times we find a wonderful power in the people to rise above their conditions. With them, however, as with other peoples, luxury, riches, comfort, bring a surfeit to initiative and the race does not accomplish so much. At various times in the early Middle Ages, particularly, we find Jewish physicians doing great work and obtaining precious acknowledgment for it in spite of the most discouraging conditions. Later it is not unusual to find that there has been a degeneration into mere money-making as the result of opportunity and consequent ease and luxury. At a number of times, however, both in Christian and in Moham medan countries, great Jewish physicians arose whose names have come to us and with whom every student of medicine who wants to know something about the details of the course of medical history must be familiar. There are men among them who must be considered among the great lights of medicine, significant makers always of the art and also in nearly all cases of the science of medicine.

A little consideration of the history of the Jewish people and their great documents eliminates any surprise there may be with regard to their interest in medicine and successful pursuit of it during the Middle Ages. The two great collections of Hebrew documents, the Old Testament and the Talmud, contain an immense amount of material with reference to medical problems of many kinds. Both of these works are especially interesting because of what they have to say of preventive medicine and with regard to the recognition of disease. Our prophylaxis and diagnosis are important scientific departments of medicine dependent on observation rather than on theory. While therapeutics has wandered into all sorts of absurdities, the advances made in prophylaxis and in diagnosis have always remained valuable, and though at times they have been forgotten, re-discovery only emphasizes the value of preceding work. It is because of what they contain with regard to these two important medical subjects that the Old Testament and the Talmud are landmarks in the history of medicine as well as of religion.

Baas, in his "Outlines of the History of Medicine," says: "It corresponds to the reality in both the actual and chronological point of view to consider the books of Moses as the foundation of sanitary science. The more we have learned about sanitation in the prophylaxis of disease and in the prevention of contagion in the modern time, the more have we come to appreciate highly the teachings of these old times on such subjects. Moses made a masterly exposition of the knowledge necessary to prevent contagious disease when he laid down the rules with regard to leprosy, first as to careful differentiation, then as to isolation, and finally as to disinfection after it had come to be sure that cure had taken place. The great lawgiver could insist emphatically that the keeping of the laws of God not only was good for a man's soul but also for his body."

With this tradition familiarly known and deeply studied by the mass of the Hebrew people, it is no surprise to find that when the next great Hebrew development of religious writing came in the Talmud during the earlier Middle Ages, that also contains much with regard to medicine, not a little of which is so close to absolute truth as never to be out of date. Friedenwald, in his "Jewish Physicians and the Contributions of the Jews to the Science of Medicine," a lecture delivered before the Gratz College of Philadelphia fifteen years ago, summed up from Baas' "History of Medicine" the instructions in the Talmud with regard to health and disease. The summary represents so much more of genuine knowledge of medicine and surgery than might be expected at the early period at which it was written, during the first and second century of our era, that it seems well to quote it at some length.

> "Fever was regarded as nature's effort to expel morbific matter and restore health; which is a much safer interpretation of fever, from a practical point of view, than most of the

theories bearing on this point that have been taught up to a very recent period. They attributed the halting in the hind legs of a lamb to a callosity formed around the spinal cord. This was a great advance in the knowledge of the physiology of the nervous system. An emetic was recommended as the best remedy for nausea. In many cases no better remedy is known to-day. They taught that a sudden change in diet was injurious, even if the quality brought by the change was better. That milk fresh from the udder was the best. The Talmud describes jaundice and correctly ascribes it to the retention of bile, and speaks of dropsy as due to the retention of urine. It teaches that atrophy or rupture of the kidneys is fatal. Induration of the lungs (tuberculosis) was regarded as incurable. Suppuration of the spinal cord had an early, grave meaning. Rabies was known. The following is a description given of the dog's condition: 'His mouth is open, the saliva issues from his mouth; his ears drop; his tail hangs between his legs; he runs sideways, and the dogs bark at him; others say that he barks himself, and that his voice is very weak. No man has appeared who could say that he has seen a man live who was bitten by a mad dog.' The description is good, and this prognosis as to hydrophobia in man has remained unaltered till in our day when Pasteur published his startling revelation. The anatomical knowledge of the Talmudists was derived chiefly from dissection of the animals. As a very remarkable piece of practical anatomy for its very early date is the procuring of the skeleton from the body of a prostitute by the process of boiling, by Rabbi

Ishmael, a physician, at the close of the first century. He gives the number of bones as 252 instead of 232. The Talmudists knew the origin of the spinal cord at the foramen magnum and its form of termination; they described the œsophagus as being composed of two coats; they speak of the pleura as the double covering of the lungs; and mention the special coat of fat about the kidneys. They had made progress in obstetrics; described monstrosities and congenital deformities; practised version, evisceration, and Cæsarian section upon the dead and upon the living mother. A. H. Israels has clearly shown in his 'Dissertatio Historico-Medica Inauguralis' that Cæsarian section, according to the Talmud, was performed among the Jews with safety to mother and child. The surgery of the Talmud includes a knowledge of dislocation of the thigh bone, contusions of the skull, perforation of the lungs, œsophagus, stomach, small intestines, and gall bladder; wounds of the spinal cord, windpipe, of fractures of the ribs, etc. They described imperforate anus and how it was to be relieved by operation. Chanina Ben Chania inserted natural and wooden teeth as early as the second century, C. E."

There is a famous summing up of the possibilities of life and happiness in the Talmud that has been often quoted—its possible wanting in gallantry being set down to the times in which it was written. "Life is compatible with

> any disease, provided the bowels remain open; any kind of pain, provided the heart remain unaffected; any kind of uneasiness, provided the head is not attacked; all manner of evils, except it be a bad woman."

There are many other interesting suggestions in the Talmud. Sometimes they have come to be generally accepted in the modern time, sometimes they are only curious notions that have not, however, lost all their interest. The crucial incision for carbuncle is a typical example of the first class and the suggestion of the removal of superfluous fat from within the abdomen or in the abdominal wall itself by operation is another. That they had some idea of the danger of sepsis may be gathered from the fact that they suspected iron surgical instruments and advised the use of others of less enduring character.

The Talmud itself was indeed a sort of encyclopedia in which was gathered knowledge of all kinds from many sources. It was not particularly a book of medicine, though it contains so many medical ideas. In many parts of it the authors' regard for science is emphatically expressed. Landau, in his "History of Jewish Physicians," closes his account of the Talmud with this paragraph:

> "I conclude this brief review of Talmudic medicine with some reference to how high the worth of science was valued in this much misunderstood work. In one place we have the expression 'occupation with science means more than sacrifice.' In another 'science is more than priesthood and kingly dignity.'"[4]

After all this of national tradition in medicine before and after Christ, it is only what we might quite naturally expect to find, that there is scarcely a century of the Middle Ages which does not contain at least one great Jewish physician and sometimes there are more. Many of these men made distinct contributions to medical science and their names have been held in high estimation ever since. Perhaps I should say that they were held in high estimation until that neglect of historical studies which characterized the eighteenth century developed, and that there has been a reawakening of interest in our time. We forget this curious decadence of the later seventeenth and eighteenth centuries which did so much to obscure history and especially the history of the sciences. Fortunately the scholars of the sixteenth and early seventeenth centuries accomplished successfully the task of printing many of the books of these old-time physicians and secured their publication in magnificent editions. These were bought eagerly by scholars and libraries all over Europe in spite of the high price they commanded in that era of slow, laborious printing. The Renaissance exhibits some of its most admirable qualities in its reverence for these old workers in science and above all for the careful preparation by its scholars of the text of these first editions of old-time physicians. The works have often been thus literally preserved for us, for some of them at least would have disappeared among the vicissitudes of the intervening time, most of which was anything but favorable to the preservation of old-time works, no matter what their content or value.

During the second and third centuries of our era, while the Talmudic writings were taking shape, three great Jewish physicians came into prominence. The first of them, Chanina, was a contemporary of Galen. According to tradition, as we have said, he inserted both natural and artificial teeth before the close of the second century. The two others were Rab or Raw and Samuel. Rab has the distinction of having studied his anatomy from the human body. According to tradition he did not hesitate to spend large sums of money in order to procure subjects for dissection. At this time it is very doubtful whether Galen, though only of the preceding generation, ever had the opportunity to study more than animals or, at most, a few human bodies. Samuel, the third of the group, was an intimate friend of Rab's, perhaps a disciple, and his fame depends rather on his practice of medicine than of research in medical science. He was noted for his practical development of two specialties that cannot but seem to us rather distant from each other. His reputation as a skilful obstetrician was only surpassed by the estimation in which he was held as an oculist. He seems to have turned to astronomy as a hobby, and was highly honored for his knowledge of this science. Probably there is nothing commoner in the story of great Jewish physicians than their successful pursuit of some scientific subject as a hobby and reaching distinction in it. Their surplus intellectual energy needed an outlet besides their vocation, and they got a rest by turning to some other interest, often accomplishing excellent results in it. Like most great students with a hobby, the majority of them were long-lived. Their lives are a lesson to a generation that fears intellectual overwork.

During the fourth century we have a number of very interesting traditions with regard to a great Jewish physician, Abba Oumna, to whom patients flocked from all over the world. He seems particularly to have been anxious to make his services available to the scholars of his time. He looked upon them as brothers in spirit, fellow-laborers whose investigations were as important as his own and whose labors for mankind he hoped to extend by the helpfulness of his profession. In order that it might be easy for them to come to him without feeling abashed by their poverty, and yet so that they might pay him anything that they thought they were able to, he hung up a box in his anteroom in which each patient might deposit whatever he felt able to give. His kindliness towards men became the foundation for many legends. Needless to say he was often imposed upon, but that seems to have made no difference to him, and he went on straightforwardly doing what he thought he ought to do, regardless of the devious ways of men, even those whom he was generously assisting. While we do not know much of his scientific medicine, we do know that he was a fine example of a practitioner of medicine on the highest professional lines.

With the foundation of the school at Djondisabour in Arabistan or Khusistan by the Persian monarch Chosroes, some Jewish physicians come into prominence as teachers, and this is one of the first important occasions in history when they teach side by side with Christian colleagues. Djondisabour seems distant from us now, lying as it does in the province just above the head of the Persian Gulf, and it is a little hard to understand its becoming a centre of culture and education, yet according to well-grounded historical traditions students flocked here from all parts of the world, and its medical instruction particularly became famous. According to the documents and traditions that we possess, clinical teaching was the most significant feature of the school work and made it famous. As a consequence graduates from here were deemed fully qualified to become professors in other institutions and were eagerly sought by various medical schools in the East.

With the rise of the strong political power of the Mohammedans enough of peace came to the East at least to permit the cultivation of arts and sciences to some extent again, and then at once the eminence of Jewish physicians, both as teachers and practitioners of medicine, once more becomes manifest. The first of the race who comes into prominence is Maser Djawah Ebn Djeldjal, of Basra. To him we owe probably more than to anyone else the preservation of old scientific writings and the cultivation of arts and sciences by the Mohammedans. He prevailed on Caliph Moawia I, whose physician he had become, to cause many foreign works, and especially those written in Greek, to be translated into Arabic. He seems to have taken a large share of the labor of the translation on himself and prevailed upon his pupil, the son of Moawia, to translate some works on chemistry. The translation for which Maser Djawah is best known is that of the Pandects of Haroun, a physician of Alexandria. The translation of this work was made toward the end of the seventh century. Unfortunately the "Pandects" has not come down to us, either in original or translation, but we have fragments of the translation preserved by Rhazes, the distinguished Arabian medical writer and physician of the ninth century, and there seems no doubt that it contained the first good description of smallpox, a chapter in medicine that is often—though incorrectly—attributed to Rhazes himself. Rhazes quoted Maser Djawah freely and evidently trusted his declarations implicitly.

The succeeding Caliphs of the first Arabian dynasty did not exhibit the same interest in education, and above all in science, that characterized Moawia. Political ambition and the desire for military glory seem to have filled up their thoughts and perhaps they had not the good fortune to fall under the influence of physicians so wise and learned as Maser Djawah. More probably, however, they themselves lacked interest. Toward the end of the seventh century they were succeeded by the Abbassides. Almansor, the second Caliph of this dynasty, was attacked by a dangerous disease and sent for a physician of the Nestorian school. After his restoration to health he became a liberal patron of science and especially medical science. The new city of Bagdad, which had become the capital of the realm of the Abbassides, was enriched by him with a large number of works on medicine, which he caused to be translated from the Greek. He did not confine himself to medicine, however, but also brought about translations of works with regard to other sciences. One of these, astronomy, was a favorite. He made it a particular point to search out and encourage the translation of such books as had not previously been translated from Greek into Arabic. While he provided a translation of Ptolemy he also had translations made of Aristotle and Galen.

It is not surprising, then, that the school of Bagdad became celebrated. Jewish physicians seem to have been most prominent in its foundation, and the most distinguished product of it is Isaac Ben Emran, almost as celebrated as a philosopher as he is as a physician. One of his expressions with regard to the danger of a patient having two physicians whose opinions disagree with regard to his illness has been deservedly preserved for us. Zeid, an Emir of one of the chief cities of the Arabs in Barbary, fell ill of a tertian fever and called Isaac and another physician in consultation. Their opinions were so widely in disaccord that Isaac refused to prescribe anything, and when the Emir, who had great confidence in him, demanded the reason, he replied, "disagreement of two physicians is more deadly than a tertian fever." This Isaac, who is said to have died in 799, is the great Jewish physician, one of the most important members of the profession in the eighth century. His principal work was with regard to poisons and the symptoms caused by them. This is often quoted by medical writers in the after time.

The prominent Jewish physician of the ninth century was Joshua Ben Nun. Haroun al-Raschid, whose attempts to secure justice for his people are the subject of so much legendary lore, and whose place in history may be best recalled by the fact that he is a contemporary of Charlemagne, was particularly interested in medicine. He founded the city of Tauris as a memorial of the cure of his wife. He was a generous patron of the school of Djondisabour and established a medical school also at Bagdad. He provided good salaries for the professors, insisted on careful examinations, and raised the standard of medical education for a time to a noteworthy degree. The greatest teacher of this school at Bagdad was Joshua Ben Nun, sometimes known as the Rabbi of Seleucia. His teaching attracted many students to Bagdad and his fame as one of the great practitioners of medicine of this time brought many patients. Among his disciples was John Masuée, whose Arabian name is so different, Yahia Ben Masoviah, that in order to avoid confusion in reading it is important to know both. Almost better known, perhaps, at this time was Abu Joseph Jacob Ben Isaac Kendi. Fortunately for the after time, these men devoted themselves not only to their own observations and writings but made a series of valuable translations. Joshua Ben Nun seems to have been particularly zealous in this matter, following the example of Maser Djawah of Basra.

Bagdad then became a centre for Arabian culture. Mahmoud, one of Haroun's successors, provided in Bagdad a refuge for the learned men of the East who were disturbed by the wars and troubles of the time. He became a liberal patron of literature and education. When the Emperor Michael III of Constantinople was conquered in battle, one of the obligations imposed upon him was to send many camel loads of books to Bagdad, and Aristotle and Plato were studied devotedly and translated into Arabic. The era of culture affected not only the capital but all the cities, and everywhere throughout the Arabian empire schools and academies sprang up. We have records of them at Basra, Samarcand, Ispahan. From here the thirst for education spread to the other cities ruled by the Mohammedans, and each town became affected by it. Alexandria, the cities of the Barbary States, those of Sicily and Provence, where Moorish influences were prominent, and of distant Spain, Cordova, Seville, Toledo, Granada, Saragossa, all took up the rivalry for culture which made this a glorious period in the history of the intellectual life.

Already, in the chapter on "Great Physicians in Early Christian Times," I have pointed out that many of the teachers of the Arabs were Christian physicians. Here it is proper to emphasize the other important factor in Arabian medicine, the Jewish physicians, who influenced the great Arabian rulers, and were the teachers of the Arabs in medicine and science generally. These Christian and Jewish physicians particularly encouraged the translation of the works of the great Greek physicians and thus kept the Greek medical tradition from dying out. It is not until the end of the ninth, or even the beginning of the tenth, century that we begin to have important contributors to medicine from among the Arabs themselves. Even at this time they have distinguished rivals among Jewish physicians. Indeed these acquired such a reputation that they became the physicians to monarchs and even high ecclesiastics, and we find them nearly everywhere throughout Europe. Their success was so great that it is not surprising that after a time the vogue of the Jewish physicians should have led to jealousy of them and to the passage of laws and decrees limiting their sphere of activity.

The great Jewish physician of the ninth century was Isaac Ben Soliman, better known as Isaac el Israili, and who is sometimes spoken of as d'Israeli. He was a pupil of Isaac Ben Amram the younger, probably a grandson of another Isaac Ben Amram, who, after having become famous in Bagdad, went to Cairo and became the physician of the Emir Zijadeth III. The younger Isaac established a school, and it was with him that Israeli obtained his introduction to medicine. He practised first as an oculist and then became body-physician to the Sultan of Morocco. Because of the sympathy of his character and his unselfishness he acquired great popularity. Hyrtl refers to him respectfully as "that scholarly son of Israel." Curiously enough, considering racial feeling in the matter, he never married, and when asked why he had not, and whether he did not think that he might regret it, he replied, "I have written four books through which my memory will be better preserved than it would be by descendants." The four books are his "Treatise on Fevers," his "Treatise on Simple Medicines and Ailments," a treatise on the "Elements," and a treatise "On the Urine." Besides these, we have from him shorter works, "On the Pulse," "On Melancholy," and "On Dropsy." His hope with regard to his fame from these works was fulfilled, for they were printed as late as 1515 at Leyden, and Sprengel declared them the best compendium of simple remedies and diet that we have from the Arabian times. One of his translators into Latin has called him the monarch of physicians.

Some of his maxims are extremely interesting in the light of modern notions on the same subjects. He declared emphatically that "the most important duty of the physician is to prevent illness." "Most patients get better without much help from the physician by the power of nature." He emphasized his distrust of using many medicines at the same time in the hope that some of them would do good. He laid it down as a rule: "Employ only one medicine at a time in all your cases and note its effects carefully." He was as wise with regard to medical ethics as therapeutics. He advised a young physician, "Never speak unfavorably of other physicians. Every one of us has his lucky and unlucky hours." It is pleasant to learn that the old gentleman lived to fill out a full hundred years of life, and that in his declining years he was surrounded by the good will and the affection of many who had learned to know his precious qualities of heart and mind. More than of any other class of physicians do we find the large human sympathies of the Jewish physicians of the Middle Ages praised by their contemporaries and succeeding generations.

During the next centuries a number of Jewish physicians became prominent, though none of them until Maimonides impressed themselves deeply upon the medical life of their own and succeeding centuries. Very frequently they were the physicians to royal personages. Zedkias, for instance, was the physician to Louis the Pious and later to his son Charles the Bald. His reputation as a physician was great enough to give him the popular estimation of a magician, but it did not save him from the accusation of having poisoned Charles when that monarch died suddenly. There seem to be no good grounds, however, for the accusation. There were a number of schools of medicine, in Sicily and the southern part of Italy, in which Jewish, Arabian, and Christian physicians taught side by side. One of these teachers was Jude Sabatai Ben Abraham, usually known by the name of Donolo, who was famous both as a writer on medicine and on astronomy. Donolo studied and probably taught at Tarentum, and there were similar schools at Palermo, at Bari, and then later on the mainland at Salerno. The foundation of Salerno, in which Jewish physicians also took part, we shall discuss later in the special chapter devoted to that subject.

One of the great translators whose work meant very much for the medical science of his own and succeeding generations was the distinguished Jewish physician, Faradj Ben Salim, sometimes spoken of as Farachi Faragut or Ferrarius, who was born at Girgenti in Sicily. He made his medical studies in Salerno and did his work under the patronage of Charles of Anjou towards the end of the thirteenth century. His greatest work is the translation of the whole of the "Continens" of Rhazes. The translation is praised as probably the best of its time made in the Middle Ages. Faradj came at the end of a great century, when the intellectual life of Europe had reached a high power of expression, and it is not surprising that he should have proved equal to his environment. This translation has also some additions made by Faradj himself, notably a glossary of Arabian names.

In Spain also Jewish physicians rose to distinction. The most distinguished in the tenth century was Chasdai Ben Schaprut. Like many other of the great physicians of this time, he had studied astronomy as well as the medical sciences. He became the physician of the Caliph Abd-er-Rahman III of Cordova. He seems also to have exercised some of the functions of Prime Minister to the Caliph, and took advantage of diplomatic relations between his sovereign and the Byzantine Emperor to obtain some works of Dioscorides. These he translated into Arabian with the help of a Greek monk, whom he seems also to have secured through the diplomatic relations. Undoubtedly he did much to usher in that enthusiasm for education and study which characterized the next centuries, the eleventh and twelfth, at Cordova in Spain, when such men as Avenzoar, Avicenna, and Averroës attracted the attention of the educational world of the time. Jewish writers have sometimes claimed one of the most distinguished of these, Avenzoar himself, as a Jew, but Hyrtl and other good authorities consider him of Arabic extraction and point to the fact that his ancestors bore the name of Mohammed. This is not absolutely conclusive evidence, but because of it I have preferred to class Avenzoar among the Arabian physicians.

The one historical fact of importance for us is that everywhere in Europe at that time Jews were being accorded opportunities for the study and practice of medicine. There are local incidents of persecution, but we are not so far away from the feelings that brought these about as to misunderstand them or to think that they were anything more than local, popular manifestations. The more we know about the details of the medical history of these times the deeper is the impression of academic freedom and of opportunities for liberal education.

Much has been said about the intolerance of ecclesiastical authorities toward the Jews, and of Church decrees that either absolutely forbade their practice of the medical profession and their devotion to scientific study, or at least made these pursuits much more difficult for them than for others. Of course it has to be conceded, even by those who most insistently urge the existence of formal legislation in the matter, that in spite of these decrees and intolerance and opposition, Jews continued to practise medicine and to be the chosen physicians of kings and even of high ecclesiastical dignitaries, as well indeed of the Popes themselves. This, it is usually declared, must be attributed to the surpassing skill of the Jewish physicians, causing men to overcome their prejudices and override even their own legal regulations. There is no doubt at all about the skill of Jewish physicians at many times during the Middle Ages. There is no doubt also of the sentiment of opposition that often developed between the Christian peoples and the Jews. Any excuse is good enough to justify men, to themselves at least, in putting obstacles in the paths of those who are more successful than they are themselves. Religion often became a cloak for ill-will and persecution.

The state of affairs that has been presumed however, according to which laws and decrees were being constantly issued forbidding the practice of medicine to Jews by the ecclesiastical authorities, while at the same time they themselves and those who were nearest to them were employing Jewish physicians, is an absurdity that on the face of it calls for investigation of the conditions and from its very appearance would indicate that the ordinary historical assumption in the matter must be wrong.

I have been at some pains, then, to try to find out just what were the conditions in Europe with regard to the practice of medicine by the Jews. There is no doubt that at Salerno, where the influence of the Benedictines was very strong and where the influence of the Popes and the ecclesiastical authorities was always dominant, full liberty of studying and teaching was from the earliest days allowed to the Jews. Down at Montpellier it seems clear that Jewish physicians had a large part in the foundation of the medical school, and continued for several centuries to be most important factors in the maintenance of its reputation and the upbuilding of that fame which draw students from even distant parts of Europe to this medical school of the south of France. During the ninth, tenth, eleventh, and twelfth centuries Jewish physicians were frequently in attendance on kings and the higher nobility, on bishops and archbishops, cardinals, and even Popes. Every now and then the spirit of intolerance among the populace was aroused, and occasionally the death of some distinguished patient while in a Jewish physician's hands was made the occasion for persecution. We must not forget, after all, that even as late as Elizabeth's time, when Shakespeare wrote "The Merchant of Venice," he was taking advantage of the popular sentiment aroused by the execution of Lopez, the Queen's physician, for a real or supposed participation in a plot against her Majesty's life. Shylock was presented the next season for the sake of adventitious popularity that would thus accrue to the piece. The character was played so as to depict all the worst traits of the Jew, and was scornfully laughed at at every representation. This is an index of the popular feeling of the time. Bitter intolerance of the Jew has continued. Down almost to our own time the Ghettos have existed in Europe, and popular tumults against them continue to occur. Quite needless to say, these do not depend on Christianity, but on defective human nature.

During the Middle Ages the best possible criterion of the attitude of the Church authorities towards the Jews is to be found in the legislation of Pope Innocent III. He is the greatest of the Popes of the Middle Ages; he shaped the policy of the Church more than any other; his influence was felt for many generations after his own time. His famous edict with regard to them was well known: "Let no Christian by violence compel them to come dissenting or unwilling to Baptism. Further, let no Christian venture maliciously to harm their persons without a judgment of the civil power or to carry off their property or change their good customs which they have hitherto in that district which they inhabit." Innocent himself and several of his predecessors and successors are known to have had Jewish physicians. Example speaks even louder than precept, and the example of such men must have been a wonderful advertisement for the Jewish physicians of the time.

Besides Innocent III, many of the Popes of the twelfth and thirteenth centuries issued similar decrees as to the Jews. It may be recalled that this was the time when the Papacy was most powerful in Europe and when its decrees had most weight in all countries. Alexander II, Gregory IX, and Innocent IV all issued formal documents demanding the protection of the Jews, and especially insisting that they must not be forced to receive Baptism nor disturbed in the celebration of their festivals. Clement VI did the same thing in the next century, and even offered them a refuge from persecution throughout the rest of France at Avignon. Distinguished Jewish scholars, who know the whole story from careful study, have given due credit to the Popes for all that they did for their people. They have even declared that]if the Jews were not exterminated in many of the European countries it was because of the protection afforded by the Church. We have come to realize in recent years that persecution of the Jews is not at all a religious matter, but is due to racial prejudice and jealousy of their success by the peoples among whom they settle. All sorts of pretexts are given for this persecution at all times. Formal Church documents and the personal activities of the responsible Church officials show that during the Middle Ages the Church was a protector and not a persecutor of the Jews.

There is abundant historical authority for the statement that the Popes were uniformly beneficent in their treatment of the Jews. In order to demonstrate this there is no need to quote Catholic historians, for non-Catholics have been rather emphatic in bringing it out. Neander, the German Protestant historian, for instance, said:

> "It was a ruling principle with the Popes after the example of their great predecessor, Gregory the Great, to protect the Jews in the rights which had been conceded to them. When the banished Popes of the twelfth century returned to Rome, the Jews went forth in their holiday garments to meet them, bearing before them the 'thora,' and Innocent II, on an occasion of this sort, blessed them."

English non-Catholic historians can be quoted to the same effect. The Anglican Dean Milman, for instance, said: "Of all European sovereigns, the Popes, with some

> exceptions, have pursued the most humane policy towards the Jews. In Italy, and even in Rome, they have been more rarely molested than in the other countries."

Hallam has expressed himself to the same effect, especially as regards the protection afforded to the Jew by the laws of the Church from the injustice of those around him. Laws sometimes fail of their purpose and the persecuting spirit of the populace is often hard to control, but everything that the central authority could do to afford protection was done and essential justice was enshrined in the Church laws.

Prominent ecclesiastics would naturally follow the lines laid down by their Papal superiors. The attitude of those whose lives mark epochs in the history of Christianity and who had more to do almost with the shaping of the policy of the Church at many times than the Popes themselves, can be quoted readily to this same effect. Neander has called particular attention to St. Bernard's declarations with regard to the evils that would follow any tolerance of such an abuse as the persecution of the Jews.

> "The most influential men of the Church protested against such un-Christian fanaticism. When the Abbot Bernard of Clairvaux was rousing up the spirit of the nations to embark in the second crusade, and issued for this purpose, in the year 1146, his letters to the Germans (East Franks), he at the

> same time warned them against the influence of those enthusiasts who strove to inflame the fanaticism of the people. He declaimed against the false zeal, without knowledge, which impelled them to murder the Jews, a people who ought to be allowed to live in peace in the country."

But it has been said that there are decrees against Jewish physicians, issued especially in the south of France, by various councils and synods of the Church. Attention needs to be called at once to the fact that these are entirely local regulations and have nothing to do with the attitude of the Church as a whole, but represent what the ecclesiastical authorities of a particular part of the country deem necessary for some special reason in order to meet local conditions. Indeed at the end of the thirteenth and the early fourteenth century, when these decrees were being issued in France, full liberty was allowed in Italy, and there were no restrictions either as to medical practice or education founded on adhesion to Judaism.

What need to be realized in order to understand the issuance of certain local ecclesiastical regulations forbidding Jews to practise medicine are the special conditions which developed in France at this time. Many Jews had emigrated from Spain to France, and the reputation acquired by Jewish physicians at Montpellier led to a number of the race taking up the practice of medicine without any further qualification than the fact that they were Jews. That gave them a reputation for curative powers of itself because of the fame of some

Jewish doctors and their employment by the nobility and the highest ecclesiastics. It was hard to regulate these wandering physicians. As a consequence of this, the faculty at Paris, always jealous of its own rights and those of its students, at the beginning of the fourteenth century absolutely forbade Jews from practising on Christian patients within its jurisdiction. Of course the faculty of the University of Paris was dominated by ecclesiastical authorities. The medical school was, however, almost entirely independent of ecclesiastical influence, and was besides largely responsible for this decree. It was felt that something had to be done to stop the evil that had arisen and the charlatanry and quackery which was being practised. This was, however, rather an attempt to regulate the practice of medicine and keep it in the hands of medical school graduates than an example of intolerance towards the Jews. Practically no Jews had graduated at its university, Montpellier being their favorite school, and Paris was not a little jealous of its rights to provide for physicians from the northern part of France. We have not got away from manifestations of that spirit even yet, as our non-reciprocating state medical laws show.

During the next quarter of a century decrees not unlike those of the University of Paris were issued in the south of France, especially in Provence and Avignon. Anyone who knows the conditions which existed in the south of France at this time with regard to medical practice will be aware that a number of attempts were made by the ecclesiastical authorities just at this time to regulate the practice of medicine. Great abuses had crept in. Almost anyone who wished could set up as a physician, and those who were least fitted were often best able to secure a large number of patients by their cleverness, their knowledge of men, and their smooth tongues. The bishops of various dioceses met, and issued decrees forbidding anyone from practising medicine unless he was a graduate of the medical school of the neighboring University of Montpellier. After a time it was found that the greatest number of violators of these decrees were Jews. Accordingly special regulations were made against them. They happen to be ecclesiastical regulations, because no other authority at that time claimed the right to regulate medical education and the practice of medicine.

What is sure is that many Jewish physicians reached distinction under Christian as well as Arabian rulers at all times during the Middle Ages. It would be quite impossible in the limited space at command here to give any adequate mention of what was accomplished by these Jewish physicians, whose names we have scarcely been able to more than catalogue, nor of the place they hold in their times. As the physicians of rulers, their influence for culture and the cultivation of science was extensive, and as a rule they stood for what was best and highest in education. The story of one of them, who is generally known in the Christian world at least, Maimonides, given in some detail, may serve as a type of these Jewish physicians of the Middle Ages. He lived just before the flourishing period of university life in the thirteenth century brought about that wonderful development of medicine and surgery in the west of Europe that meant so much for the final centuries of the Middle Ages. His works influenced not a little the great thinkers and teachers whose own writings were to be the foundations of education for several centuries after their time. Maimonides was well known in the Western universities. Though his life had been mainly spent in the East, and he died there, there was scarcely a distinguished scholar of Europe who was not acquainted directly or indirectly with his works, and the greater the reputation of the scholar, as a rule, the more he knew of Maimonides, Moses Ægyptæus, as he was called, and the more frequently he referred to his writings.

IV

MAIMONIDES

The life of one of the great Jewish physicians, who has come to be known in history as Maimonides, is of such significance in medical biography that he deserves to have a separate sketch. Born in Spain, his life was lived in the East, where his connection as royal physician with the great Sultan Saladin of Crusades fame made his influence widely felt. He is a type of the broadly educated man, conversant with the culture of his time and of the past, knowing much besides medicine, who has so often impressed himself deeply on medical practice. While the narrow specialists in each generation, the men who are quite sure that they are curing the special ills of men to which they devote themselves, have always felt that whatever of progress there was in any given time was due to them, they occupy but little space as a rule in the history of medicine. The men who loom large were the broad-minded, humanely sympathetic, deeply educated physicians, who treated men and their ills rather than their ills without due consideration of the individual, and who not only relieved the discomfort of their patients and greatly lessened human suffering, and added to the sum of human happiness in their time, but also left precious deeply significant lessons for succeeding generations of their profession. Hippocrates, Galen, Sydenham, Auenbrugger, Morgagni, these are representatives of this great class, and Maimonides must be considered one of them.

Moses Ben Maimum, whose Arabic name was Abu Amran Musa Ben Maimum Obaid Alla el-Cordovi, who was called by his Jewish compatriots Ramban or Rambam, was born at Cordova in Spain, on the 30th of March in 1135 or 1139, the year is in doubt. It might not seem of much import now after nearly eight centuries, but not a little ink is spilt over it yet by devoted biographers.

We are rather prone to think in our time that the conditions in which men were born and reared before what we are pleased to call modern times, and, above all, in the Middle Ages, must have made a distinct handicap for their intellectual development. Most of us are quite sure that the conditions in medieval cities were eminently unsuited for the stimulation of the intellect, for incentive to art impulse, for uplift in the intellectual life, or for any such broad interest in what has been so well called the humanities — the humanizing things that lift us above animal necessities — as would make for genuinely liberal education. We are likely to be set in the opinion that the environment of the growing youth of an old-time city, especially so early as the middle of the twelfth century, was poor and sordid. The cares of the citizens are presumed to have been mainly for material concerns, and, indeed, mostly for the wants of the body. They were only making a start on the way from barbarism to something like our glorious culmination of civilization. As "the heirs to all the ages in the foremost files of time" we are necessarily far in advance of them, and we are only sorry that they did not have the opportunity to live to see our day and enjoy the benefits of the evolution of humanity that is taking place during the eight centuries that have elapsed.

As a matter of fact, there was much more of abiding profound interest in real civilization in many a medieval city, much more general appreciation of art, much more breadth of intelligence and sympathy with what we call the humanities, than in most of our large cities. The large city, as we know it, is eminently a discourager of breadth of intelligence. Specialism in the various phases of money-making obscures culture. Maimonides, born in Cordova, was brought up amid surroundings that teemed with incentives of every kind to the development of intelligence, of artistic taste, and everything that makes for cultivation of intellect rather than of interest in merely material things.

It is well said that it is hard to judge the Cordova of old by its tawdry ruins of to-day. The educated visitor still stands in awe and admiration of the great mosque which expressed the high cultivation of the Moors of this time. It is a never-ending source of wonder to Americans. The city itself has many reminders of that fine era of Moorish culture and refinement of taste and of art expression, which made it in the best sense of the word a city beautiful. The Arab invaders had found a great prosperous country which had been the most cultured province of the Roman Empire, and on this foundation they made a marvellous development. "The banks of the Guadalquivir," says Mr. S. Lane-Poole in "The Moors in Spain" (London, 1887), "were bright with marble houses, mosques, and gardens, in which the rarest flowers and trees of other countries were carefully cultivated, and the Arabs introduced their system of irrigation which the Spaniards both before and since have never equalled." The greatest beauty of the city, of course, had come, and some of it had gone, before Maimonides' time. So much remains in spite of time and war, and many unfortunate influences, that we can have some idea how beautiful it must have been in his youth seven centuries ago, and how even more beautiful in the foretime. Of the great mosque writers of travel can scarcely say enough. Mr. Lane-Poole says: "Travellers stand amazed among the forest of columns which open out apparently endless vistas on all sides. The porphyry, jasper, and marbles are still in their places; the splendid glass mosaics, which artists from Byzantium came to make, still sparkle like jewels in the walls; the daring architecture of the sanctuary, with its fantastic crossed arches, is still as imposing as ever; the courtyard is still leafy with the orange trees that prolong the vistas of columns. As one stands before the loveliness of the great mosque, the thought goes back to the days of the glories of Cordova, the palmy days of the Great Khalif, which will never return."

Of all the countries in which the Jews all down the centuries have lived there is probably none of which they have been more loud in praise than Spain. Their poets sang of it as if it were their own country; for centuries the people were happier here than probably they have been anywhere else for so long a period. Elsewhere in this book I have called attention to all that Spain meant in Europe during all the centuries from the beginning of the Roman Empire down to the end of the Middle Ages. Maimonides was fortunate in his birthplace, then, and while circumstances compelled the family to move away, this change did not come until a good effect had been produced on the mind of the growing youth. Even when persecution came, Maimonides clung to Spain with a tenacity born of deep affection and emphasized by admiration for all that she was and had been. Cordova was the jewel of the Spain of this time, and though much less than she had been in the long preceding time, when she was the birthplace of Lucan and the two Senecas, or even than what she had been in Abd-er-Rahman's days, or when she was the birthplace of Averroës, still she remained wonderfully beautiful and attractive, winning and holding the affections of men.

Maimonides' father, Maimum Ben Joseph, was a member of the Rabbinical College of Cordova, and famous for his knowledge of the Talmud. There are some writings of his on mathematics and astronomy extant. He directed the education of his son, who, like many another distinguished scholar in later life, seems to have exhibited very little talent in his early years. There is no rule in the matter. Precocity often disappoints. Genius is often dull in childhood, but there are exceptions that prove both rules. The basis of education in Spain at that time among the Jews was the Bible, the Talmud, mathematics, and astronomy, a good rounded education in literature, the basis of law, and some exact physical science. After his preliminary education at home Maimonides studied the natural sciences and medicine with Moorish teachers. Nature-study, in spite of frequent expressions that declare it new in modern times, is as old as man. He also received a grounding in philosophy as a preparation for his scientific studies. At the age of twenty-three he began the composition of a commentary on the Talmud, which he continued to work at on his journeys in Spain and in Egypt. This is considered to be one of the most important of this class of works extant, though, almost needless to say, similar writings are very numerous.

In the light of wanderings in philosophy during the centuries since, it is rather interesting to quote from that work the end of man as this Jewish philosopher of the middle of the twelfth century saw it. Recent teleological tendencies in biology add to the interest of his views. According to Maimonides, "Man is the end of the whole creation, and we have only to look to him for the reason for its existence. Every object shows the end for which it was created. The palm-trees are there to provide dates; the spider to spin her webs. All the properties of an animal or a plant are directed so as to enable it to reach its purpose in life. What is the purpose of man? It cannot lie alone in eating and drinking or yielding to passion, nor in the building of cities and the ruling of others, since these objects lie outside of him, and do not touch his essential being. Such material striving he has in common with the animal. A man is lifted from a lower to a higher condition by his reason. Only through his reason is he placed above the animals. He is the only reasonable animal. His reason enables him to understand all things, especially the Unity of God, and all knowledge and science serve only to direct man to the knowledge of God. Passions are to be subdued, since the man who yields to passion subjects his spirit to his body, and does not reveal in himself the divine power which in him lies in his reason, but is swallowed up in the ocean of matter."

Not long after Maimonides passed his twentieth year the family, consisting of the father and his two sons, Moses and David, and a daughter, moved from Cordova to Fez, compelled by Jewish persecutions. Here it is said that they had to submit to wearing the mask of Islam in order to lead a peaceful existence. This has been doubted, however, and his whole life is in flagrant contradiction with any such even apparent apostasy from the faith of his fathers. Father and son took advantage of the opportunity of intercourse with Moorish physicians and philosophers to increase their store of knowledge, but could not be content in the political and religious conditions in which they were compelled to live. About 1155, then, they went to Jerusalem, but found conditions even more intolerable there, and turned back to Egypt, where they settled down in Old Cairo. In 1166 the father died, and after this we learn that the sons made a livelihood, and even laid the foundation of a fortune, by carrying on a jewelry trade. Moses still devoted most of his time to study, while his brother did most of the business, but the brother was lost in the Indian Ocean, and with him went not only a large sum of his own money, but also much that had been entrusted to him by others. Maimonides undertook to pay off these debts and at the same time had to meet the necessities not only of himself and sister, but also of the family of his dead brother. It was then that he took up the practice of medicine and succeeded in making a great name and reputation for himself. He continued to write, however, and completed his commentary on the Talmud.

About the age of fifty Maimonides, as seems to be true of a good many men who live to old age, became rather discouraged and despondent about himself. He refers to himself in his letters and writings rather frequently as an old and ailing man. He had nearly twenty years of active life ahead of him, but he had the persuasion that comes to many that he was probably destined to an early death. His son was born shortly after this time, and that seems to have had not a little to do with brightening his life. While in Egypt Maimonides married the sister of one of the royal secretaries, who, in turn, wedded Maimonides' sister. Maimonides took on himself the education of his son, who also became a physician, though his father was not to have the satisfaction of watching his success in the practice of his chosen profession. This son, Abraham, became the physician of Malie Alkamen, the brother of Saladin, and, besides, was a physician to the hospital at Cairo. *His* son, David, the grandson of Maimonides, practised medicine also at Cairo till 1300. He in turn left two sons, Abraham and Solomon, who achieved reputation in the chosen profession of their great-grandfather.

Maimonides, after the birth of his son, became one of the busiest of practising physicians. Indeed, it is hard to understand how he had the time to do any writing in his busy life. Still less can we understand his time for teaching. He was the physician to Saladin, whose relations with Richard Cœur de Lion have made him known to English-speaking people. Every morning, as the Court physician, Maimonides went to the palace, situated half a mile away from his dwelling, and if any of the many officials and dependents that then, as now, were at Oriental courts, were ill, he stayed there for some time. As a rule he could only get back to his own home in the afternoon, and then he was, as he says himself, "almost dying with hunger." Knowing the scantiness of the Oriental breakfast, we are not surprised. There he found his waiting-room full of patients, "Jews and Mohammedans, prominent and unimportant, friends and enemies," he says himself, "a varied crowd, who are looking for my medical advice. There is scarcely time for me to get down from my carriage and wash myself and eat a little, and then until night I am constantly occupied, so that, from sheer exhaustion, I must lie down. Only on the Sabbath day have I the time to occupy myself with my own people and my studies, and so the day is away from me." What a picture it is of the busy medical teacher at all times in the world's history, yet it must not be forgotten that it is from these busy men that we have derived our most precious lessons in caring for patients rather than disease, in the art of medicine rather than medical science —and their practical lessons have been valuable long after the fine-spun theories of the scientist that took so long to elaborate have been placed definitely in the lumber room.

His reputation as a writer on medical topics is not as great as that which has been accorded him for his writings on philosophy and in Talmudic literature, but he well deserves a place among the great practical masters of medicine, as well as high rank among the physicians of his time. There is little that is original in his writing, but his thoroughgoing common sense, his wide knowledge, and his discriminating, eclectic faculty make his writings of special value. As might have been expected, the Aphorisms of Hippocrates attracted his attention, and, besides, he wrote a series of aphorisms of his own. The most interesting of his writings, however, is a series of letters on dietetics written for the son of his patron Saladin. The young prince seems to have suffered from one of the neurotic conditions that so often develop in those who have their lives all planned for them, and little incentive to do things for themselves. The main portion of his complaints centred, as in the case of many another individual of leisure, in disturbances of digestion. Besides, he suffered from constipation and feelings of depression. Doubtless, like many a young person of the modern time, he was quite sure that these symptoms portended some insidious organic ailment that would surely bring an early death. When fathers, having done all that there is to do, just expect their sons to enjoy the fruits of the paternal accomplishments, conditions of this kind very often develop, unless the young man proceeds to occupy himself with even more dangerous distractions than he finds in unending thought about his own feelings.

The rules of life and health that Maimonides laid down in these letters have become part of our popular medical tradition. Probably more of the ordinarily current maxims as to health have been derived from them than would possibly be suspected by anyone not familiar with them. In various forms his rules have been published a number of times. A good idea of them can be obtained from the following compendium of them, which I abbreviate from a biographical sketch of Maimonides by Dr. Oppler, which appeared in the "Deutsches Archiv für Geschichte der Medizin und Medicinische Geographie" (Bd. 2, Leipzig, 1879).

> 1. Man is bound to lead a life pleasing to God if he wants to have a healthy body, and he must hold himself far from everything that can hurt his health and accustom himself to whatever renews his strength. He should eat and drink only when hungry and thirsty and should be particularly careful of the regular evacuation of his bowels and of his bladder. He must not delay either of these operations, but as far as possible satisfy the inclination at once.

2. A man must not overload his stomach but be content always with something less than is necessary to make him feel quite satisfied. He should not drink much during the meal and only of water and wine mixed, taking somewhat more after digestion has begun and after digestion is completed, in moderation according to his needs. Before a man sits down to table he should note whether he has any tendency to evacuation and should make the body warm by movement and activity. After this exercise he should rest a little before taking food. It is very beneficial after work to take a bath and then the meal.

3. Food should be taken always in the sitting position. There should be no riding nor walking, nor movements of the body until digestion is finished. The man who takes a walk or any strenuous occupation immediately after eating subjects himself to serious dangers of disease.

4. Day and night should be divided into twenty-four hours. Men should sleep for eight hours, and so arrange their sleep that the end of it comes with the dawn, so that from the beginning of sleep until sunrise there should be an eight-hour interval. We should all leave our beds about the time that the sun rises.

5. During sleep a man should lie neither on his face nor on his back but on his side, the beginning of the night on his left and at the end on his right. He should not go to sleep for three or four hours after eating and should not sleep during the day.

6. Fruits that are laxative, as grapes, figs, melons, gourds, should be taken only before

meal time and not mixed with other food. It would be better to let these get into the abdominal organs and then take other food.

7. Eat what is easily digestible before what is difficult of digestion. The flesh of birds before beef and the flesh of calves before that of cows and steers. (Birds were then thought more digestible than other flesh; we have reversed the ruling. The note shows how light and digestible their flesh was considered and the reason therefor.)

8. In summer eat cooling food, acids, and no spices. In winter, on the contrary, eat warming foods, rich in spices, mustard, and other heating substances. In cold and warm climates one should eat according to the climatic conditions.

9. There are certain harmful foods that should be avoided. Large salt fish, old cheese, old pickled meat, young new wine, evil-smelling and bitter foods are often poisonous. There are also some which are less harmful, but are not to be recommended as ordinary nutritive materials. Large fish, cheese, milk more than twenty-four hours after milking, the flesh of old oxen, beans, peas, unleavened bread, sauerkraut, onions, radishes and the like. These are to be taken only in small quantities and only in the winter time and they should be avoided in the summer. Beans and lentils are to be recommended neither in winter nor summer.

10. As a rule one should avoid the eating of tree fruits, or not eat much of them, especially when they are dry and even less when they are green. If they are unripe they may cause

serious damage. Johannesbrod is very harmful at all times, as are also all the sour fruits, and only small amounts of them should be eaten in summer or in warm countries.

11. The fruits that are to be recommended dry as well as fresh, are figs, grapes, and almonds. These may be eaten as one has the appetite for them, but one should not accustom himself to eat them much, though they are healthier than all other fruits.

12. Honey and wine are not good for children, though they are beneficial for older people, especially in winter. In summer one-third less of them should be eaten than in winter.

13. Special care should be taken to have regular movements of the bowels that carry off the impurities of the body. It is an axiom in medicine, that so long as evacuations are absent, or difficult, or require strong efforts, the individual is liable to serious disease. Every medical means should be taken to overcome constipation in order to escape its dangers. For this purpose young people should be given salty food, materials that have been soaked in olive oil, salt itself, or certain vegetable soups with olive oil and salt. Older people should take honey mixed with warm water early in the morning and four hours later should take their breakfast. This proceeding should be followed up from one to four days until the constipation is overcome.

14. Another axiom of medicine is that so long as a man is able to be active and vigorous, does not eat until he is over-full, and does not suffer from constipation, he is not liable to disease. Even such men, however, are much

safer if they do not take food that may disagree with them.

15. Whoever gives himself up to inactivity, or puts off evacuations of the bowels, or suffers from constipation, will be sure to suffer from many diseases and will see his strength disappear even should he eat the best food in the world and make use of all the remedies that physicians have. Immoderate eating is a poison for men and the cause of many diseases which attack them. Most diseases come from either eating too much or partaking of unsuitable food. That was what Solomon meant with his proverb: "He who puts a guard over his mouth and his tongue protects himself from many evils," that is to say, whoever protects his mouth from the overindulgence in food and his tongue from unsuitable speech protects himself from many evils.

16. Every week at least a man should take a warm bath. One should not bathe when hungry, nor after eating until the food is digested, and bathe the whole body in warm but not too hot water and the head in hot water. Afterwards the body should be washed in lukewarm and cool water until finally cold water is used. One should pour neither cold nor even lukewarm water on the head, nor bathe in cold water in the winter time, nor when the body is tired and in perspiration. At such times the bath should be put off for a while.

17. As soon as one leaves the bath one should cover oneself, and especially cover the head, so that no draught may strike it. Even in summer,

care must be taken to observe this rule. After this one should rest for a while until the heat of the body passes off and then should go to table. If one could sleep a little just before a meal it is often very beneficial. Neither during the bath nor immediately after it should cold water be drunk, and if there is an inappeasable thirst a little wine and water or water and honey should be taken. In winter it is beneficial to rub the body with oil after the bath.

18. Venesection should not be practised frequently, for it is only meant for serious illness. It should not be permitted in winter or summer, nor during the months of April or September (the "r" months). After passing his fiftieth year an individual should abstain from venesection. Venesection should not be practised on the day when one takes a bath or goes on a journey or returns from it. On the day when it is practised less than usual should be eaten and drunk, and the patient should give himself to rest, undertake no work nor bothersome occupation, and take no walk.

19. Whoever observes these rules of life faithfully I guarantee him a long life without disease. He shall reach a good old age, and when he comes to die will not need a physician. His body will remain always strong and healthy, unless of course he has been born with a weak nature, or has had an unfortunate bringing up, or should be attacked by epidemic disease or by famine.

20. Only the healthy should keep these rules. Whoever is ill or a sufferer from any injuries, or has lost his health through bad habits, for

> him there are special rules for each disease, only to be found in the medical books. Let it be remembered that every change in a life habit is the beginning of an ailment.
>
> 21. If no physician can be secured, then ailing people may use these rules as well as the healthy.

These rules are, of course, full of the common sense of medicine that endures at all times. For the tropical climate of the Eastern countries they probably represent as good advice as could be given even at the present time. With them before us it is not surprising to find that on other subjects Maimonides was just as sensible. Perhaps in nothing is this more striking than in his complete rejection of astrology. Considering how long astrology, in the sense of the doctrine of the stars influencing human health and destinies, had dominated men's minds, and how universal was the acceptance of it, Maimonides' strong expressions show how much genius lifts itself above the popular persuasions of its time, even among the educated, and how much it anticipates subsequent knowledge.

It is well to remind ourselves that as late as the middle of the eighteenth century Mesmer's thesis on "The Influence of the Stars on Human Constitutions" was accepted by the faculty of the University of Vienna as a satisfactory evidence not only of his knowledge of medicine, but of his power to reason about it. At the end of the twelfth century Maimonides was trying to argue it out of existence on the best possible grounds. "Know, my masters," he writes, "that no man should believe anything that is not attested by one of these three sanctions:—rational proof as in mathematical science, the perception of the senses, or traditions from the prophets and learned men." His biographer in the monograph "Maimonides," published by the Jewish Publication Society of America[5], expresses his further views on the subject in compendious form, and then gives his final conclusion as follows:

> "'Works on astrology are the product of fools, who mistook vanity for wisdom. Men are inclined to believe whatever is written in a book, especially if the book be ancient; and in olden times disaster befell Israel because men devoted themselves to such idolatry instead of practising the arts of martial defence and government.' He says, that he had himself studied every extant astrological treatise, and had convinced himself that none deserved to be called scientific. Maimonides then proceeds to distinguish between astrology and astronomy, in the latter of which lies true and necessary wisdom. He ridicules the supposition that the fate of man could be dependent on the constellations, and urges that such a theory robs life of purpose, and makes man a slave of destiny. 'It is true,' he concludes, 'that you may find strange utterances in the Rabbinical literature which imply a belief in the potency of the stars at a man's nativity, but no one is justified in surrendering his own rational opinions because this or that sage erred, or because an allegorical remark is expressed literally. A man must never cast his own judgment behind him; the eyes are set in front, not in the back.'"

While Maimonides could be so positive in his opinions with regard to a subject on which he felt competent to say something, he was extremely modest with regard to many of the great problems of medicine. He often uses the expression in his writings, "I do not see how to explain this matter." He quotes with approval from a Rabbi of old who had counselled his students, "teach thy tongue to say, I do not know." In this, of course, he has given the best possible evidence of his largeness of mind and his capacity for making advance in knowledge. It is when men are ready to say, "I do not know," that progress becomes possible. It is very easy to rest in a conscious or unconscious pretence of knowledge that obscures the real question at issue. A great thinker, who lived in the century in which Maimonides died, Roger Bacon, set down as one of the four principal obstacles to advance in knowledge indeed, as *the* one of the four that hampered intellectual progress the most, the fact that men feared to say, "I do not know."

One of the most interesting features of Maimonides' career for the modern time is the influence that his writings exerted over the rising intellectual life of Europe within a half century after his death. Most people would be rather inclined to think that this Jewish author of the East would have very little influence over the thinkers and teachers of Europe within a generation after his death. He died in 1204, just at the beginning of one of the great productive centuries of humanity, perhaps one of the greatest of them all. In literature, in art, in architecture, in philosophy, and in education, this century made wonderful strides. Two of its greatest teachers, Albertus Magnus and his pupil,

Thomas Aquinas, quote from Moses Ægyptæus, the European name for Maimonides at that time, and evidently knew his writings very well. Maimonides was for them an important connecting link with the world of old Greek thought. Others of the writers and teachers of this time, as William of Auvergne, and the two great Franciscans, Alexander of Hales and Duns Scotus, were also influenced by Maimonides. In a word, the educational world of that time was much more closely united than we might think, and it did not take long for a great writer's thoughts to make themselves felt several thousand miles away. Maimonides was, then, in his own time one of the world teachers, and, in a certain sense, he must always remain that, as representing a special development of what is best in human nature.

V

GREAT ARABIAN PHYSICIANS

In order to understand the place of the Arabs in medicine and in science, a few words as to the rise of this people to political power, and then to the cultivation of literature and of science, are necessary. We hear of the Arabs as hireling soldiers fighting for others during the centuries just after Christ, and especially in connection with the story of the famous Queen Zenobia at Palmyra. After the destruction of this city we hear nothing more of them until the time of Mohammed. During these six and a half centuries there is little question of education of any kind among them except that at the end of the sixth century, the Persian King Chosroes I, who was much interested in medicine, encouraged the medical school in Djondisabour, in Arabistan, founded at the end of the fifth century by the Nestorian Christians, who continued as the teachers there until it became one of the most important schools of the East. It was here that the first Arab physicians were trained, and here that the Christian physicians who practised medicine among the Arabs were educated.

Among the Arabs themselves, before the time of Mohammed, there had been very little interest in medicine. Gurlt notes that even the physician of the Prophet himself was, according to tradition, a Christian. Mohammed's immediate successors were not interested in education, and their people mainly turned to Christian and Jewish physicians for whatever medical treatment they needed. When the Caliphs came to be rulers of the Mohammedan Empire, they took special pains to encourage the study of philosophy and medicine; though dissection was forbidden by the Koran, most of the other medical sciences, and especially botany and all the therapeutic arts, were seriously cultivated.

Until the coming of Mohammed, the Arabs had been wandering tribes, getting some fame as hireling soldiers, but now, under the influence of a feeling of community in religion, and led by the military genius of some of Mohammed's successors, whose soldiers were inspired by the religious feelings of the sect, they made great conquests. The Mohammedan Empire extended from India to Spain within a century after Mohammed's death. Carthage was taken and destroyed, Constantinople was threatened. In 661, scarcely forty years after the *hegira* or flight of Mohammed, from which good Mohammedans date their era, the capital was transferred from Medina to Damascus, to be transferred from here to Bagdad just about a century later, where it remained until the Mongols made an end of the Abbasside rulers about the middle of the thirteenth century. At the beginning the followers of Mohammed were opposed to knowledge and education of all kinds. Mohammed himself had but little. According to tradition, he could not read or write. The story told with regard to the Caliph Omar and the great library of Alexandria, seems to have a foundation in reality, though such legends usually are not to be taken literally. Certainly it represents the traditional view as to the attitude of the earlier Moslem rulers to education. Omar was asked what should be done with the more than two million volumes. He said that the books in it either agreed with the Koran, or they did not. If they agreed with it they were quite useless. If they did not, they were pernicious. In either case, they should be done away with, because there was an element of danger in them. Accordingly, the precious volumes that had been accumulating for nearly ten centuries, served, it is said, to heat the baths of Alexandria for some six months – probably the most precious fuel ever used. Fortunately for posterity, the edict was not quite as universal in its application as the story would indicate, and exceptions were made for books of science.

In the course of their conquests, however, the Mohammedan Arabs captured the Greek cities of Asia Minor. They were brought closely in contact with Greek culture, Greek literature, and Greek thought. As has always been the case, captive Greece took its captors captive. What happened to the Romans earlier came to pass also among the Arabs. Inspired by Greek philosophy, science, and literature, they became ardent devotees of science and the arts. While not inventing or discovering anything new, like the Romans they carried on the old. Damascus, Basra, Bagdad, Bokhara, Samarcand all became centres of culture and of education. Large sums were paid for Greek manuscripts, and for translations from them. Under the famous Harun al-Raschid, at the end of the eighth century, whose name is better known to us than that of any others, because of the stories of his wandering by night among his people in order to see if justice were done, three hundred scholars were sent at the cost of the Caliph to the various parts of the world in order to bring back treasures of science, and especially of geography and medicine. It is an interesting historical reflection that the Japanese and Chinese are doing the same thing now.

The Arabs were very much taken by the philosophy of Aristotle, and it became the foundation of all their education. Greek thought, as always, inspired its students to higher things. Soon everywhere in the dominions of the Caliphs, philosophy, science, art, literature, and education nourished. Medicine was taken up with the other sciences and cultivated assiduously. Freind, in his "Historia Medicinæ," says that the writings of the old Greeks which treated of medicine were saved from destruction with the other books at Alexandria, for the desire of health did not have less strength among the Arabs than among other nations. Since these books taught them how to preserve health, and were not otherwise contrary to the laws of the Prophet, that served to bring about their preservation. Freind also calls attention to the fact that grammars and books which treated of the science of language were likewise saved from destruction. Besides the library, the Arabs, after their conquest of Alexandria in the eighth century, came under the influence of the university still in existence there.

In the West, in Spain, the Arabs enjoyed the same advantages as regards contact with culture and education as their conquest of the Eastern cities and Alexandria brought them in the East. While it is not generally realized, Spain was, as we have pointed out, the province of the Roman Empire in the West that advanced most in culture before the breaking up of the Empire. The Silver Age of Latin literature owes all of its geniuses to Spain. Lucan, the

Senecas, Martial, Quintilian, are all Spaniards. Spain itself was a most flourishing province, and under the Spanish Cæsars, from the end of the first to about the end of the second century, increased rapidly in population. Spain was the leader in these prosperous times, and the tradition of culture maintained itself. When Spain became Christian the first great Christian poet, Prudentius, born about the middle of the fourth century, came from there. He has been called the Horace and Virgil of the Christians.

The coming down of the barbarians from the North disturbed Spain's prosperity and the peace and culture of her inhabitants, but it should not be forgotten that the first medieval popularization of science, a sort of encyclopedia of knowledge, the first of its kind after that of Pliny in the classical period, came from St. Isidore of Seville, a Spanish bishop.

There has been considerable tendency to insist that Spanish culture and intellectuality owe nearly all to the presence of the Moors in Spain. This can only be urged, however, by those who know nothing at all of the Spanish Cæsars, the place of Spain in the history of the Roman Empire, and the continuance of the culture that then reached a climax of expression during succeeding centuries. On the contrary, the Moors who came to Spain owe most of their tendency to devote themselves to culture and education to the state of affairs existent in Spain when they came. There is no doubt that they raised standards of education and of culture above the level to which they had sunk under the weight of the invading barbarians from the North, and Spain owes much to the wise ruling and devotion to the intellectual life of her Moorish invaders. All the factors, however, must be taken together in order to appreciate properly the conditions which developed under the Arabs in both the East and the West. The Arabs invented little that was new in science or philosophy; they merely carried on older traditions. It is for that that the modern time owes them a great debt of gratitude.

RHAZES

The most distinguished of the Arabian physicians was the man whose rather lengthy Arabian name, beginning with Abu Bekr Mohammed, finished with el-Razi, and who has hence been usually referred to in the history of medicine as Rhazes. He was born about 850 at Raj, in the Province of Chorasan in Persia. He seems to have had a liberal early education in philosophy and in philology and literature. He did not take up medicine until later in life, and, according to tradition, supported himself as a singer until he was thirty years of age. Then he devoted himself to medical studies with the ardor and the success so often noted in those whose opportunity to study medicine has been delayed. His studies were made at Bagdad, where Ibn Zein el-Taberi was his teacher. He returned to his native town and was for some time the head of the hospital there. Later he was called by the Sultan to Bagdad to take charge of the renovated and enlarged hospital of the capital. His medical career, then, is not unlike that of many another successful physician, especially of the modern time. At Bagdad he had abundant opportunities for study, and the ambition to make medicine as well as to make money and gain fame.

His studies in science were all founded on Aristotle. Though he was called the Galen of his time, and looked up to the Greek physician as his master, even the authority of Galen did not override that of the Stagirite in his estimation. One of his aphorisms is said to have been, "If Galen and Aristotle are of one mind on a subject, then surely their opinion is true. When they differ, however, it is extremely difficult for the scholar to decide which opinion should be accepted." He drew many pupils to Bagdad, and, when one knows his teaching, this is not surprising. Some of his aphorisms are very practical. While the expressions just quoted with regard to Galen and Aristotle might seem to indicate that Rhazes was absolutely wedded to authority, there is another well-known maxim of his which shows how much he thought of the value of experience and observation. "Truth in medicine," he said, "is a goal which cannot be absolutely reached, and the art of healing, as it is described in books,is far beneath the practical experience of a skilful, thoughtful physician." Some of his other medical aphorisms are worth noting. "At the beginning of a disease choose such remedies as will not lessen the patient's strength." "When you can heal by diet, prescribe no other remedy, and, where simple remedies suffice, do not take complicated ones."

Rhazes knew well the value of the influence of mind over body even in serious organic disease, and even though death seemed impending. One of his aphorisms is: "Physicians ought to console their patients even if the signs of impending death seem to be present. For the bodies of men are dependent on their spirits." He considered that the most valuable thing for the physician to do was to increase the patient's natural vitality. Hence his advice: "In treating a patient, let your first thought be to strengthen his natural vitality. If you strengthen that, you remove ever so many ills without more ado. If you weaken it, however, by the remedies that you use you always work harm." The simpler the means by which the patient's cure can be brought about, the better in his opinion. He insists again and again on diet rather than artificial remedies. "It is good for the physician that he should be able to cure disease by means of diet, if possible, rather than by means of medicine." Another of his aphorisms seems worth while quoting: "The patient who consults a great many physicians is likely to have a very confused state of mind."

Some idea of Rhazes' strenuous activity as a writer on medical subjects may be obtained from the fact that thirty-six of his works are still extant,and there are nearly two hundred others of which only the titles have been preserved. Some of these are doubtless the works of pupils and students of succeeding generations, published under his name to attract attention. His principal work is "Continens," or "Comprehensor," which owes its title to the fact that it was meant to contain the whole practice of medicine and surgery. It includes references to the writings of all previous distinguished medical writers, from Hippocrates to Honein Ben Ishac, also known as Johannitius, a Christian Arabian physician, one of Rhazes' teachers. The most frequently quoted of these authorities are Galen, Oribasius, Aëtius, and Paul of Ægina. The work, however, is not made up entirely of quotations, but contains many observations made by the author himself. Gurlt says that the foundation of the theoretic medicine of Rhazes is the system of Galen, while in practice he seems to cling more to the aphorisms of Hippocrates. He has many practical points which show that he thought for himself. For instance, in wounds of the abdomen, if the intestines are extruded and cannot be replaced, he suggests the suspension of the patient by his hands and feet in a bath in order to facilitate their return. If they do not go back readily, compresses dipped in warm wine should be used. Cancer he declares to be almost incurable. He has much to say about the bites of animals and their tendency to be poisonous, knew rabies very well, and knew also that the bites of men might have similar serious consequences.

It is impossible to give any adequate idea of the thoroughly practical character of Rhazes' medical writing in a few lines, but it may suffice to say that there is scarcely any feature of modern medicine and surgery that he does not touch, and oftener than not his touch is sure and rational and frequently much better than the advice of successors long after him in the same matters. An example or two will suffice to illustrate this. In the treatment of nasal polyps he says that whenever drug treatment of these is not successful, they should be removed with a snare made of hair. For fall of the uvula he suggests gargles, but when these fail he advises resection and cauterization. Among the affections of the tongue he numbers abscess, fissure, ulcer, cancer, ranula, shortening of the ligaments, hypertrophy, erythema of the mucous membrane, and inflammatory swelling. In general his treatment of the upper respiratory tract is much farther advanced than we might think possible at this time. He advises tracheotomy whenever there is great difficulty of respiration, and describes how it should be done. After the dyspnea has passed the edges of the wound should be brought together with sutures. It is not surprising, then, to find that the treatment of fractures and luxations is eminently practical, and, indeed, on any subject that he touches he throws practical light.

In the introduction to his edition of the works of Ambroise Paré, Malgaigne says that the first reference to a metal band in connection with trusses is to be found in Rhazes.

Hernia was, of course, one of the serious ailments that, because of its superficial character, was rather well understood, and so it is not surprising to find that much of our modern treatment of it was anticipated. The manipulations for taxis, the use of a warm bath for the relaxation of the patient by means of heat and by putting the head and feet higher than the abdomen while in the bath, and the employment of various kinds of trusses to prevent strangulation of the hernia recur over and over again, in the authors of the Middle Ages. Many of the suggestions are to be found in the early Greek authors, but subsequent writers give a certain personal expression to them which shows how much they had learned by personal observation in the employment of various methods.

Pagel, in Puschmann's "Handbook of the History of Medicine," declares that Rhazes' most important work for pure medicine is his monograph on smallpox. Its principal value is due to the fact that, though he has consulted old authorities carefully, his discussion of the disease is founded almost entirely on his own experience. His description of the various stages of the disease, of the forms of the eruption, and of the differential diagnosis, is very accurate. He compares the course of the fever with that of other fevers, and brings out exactly what constitutes the disease. His suggestions as to prognosis are excellent. Those cases, he declares, are particularly serious in which the eruption takes on a dark, or greenish, or violet color. The prognosis is also unfavorable for those cases which, having considerable fever, have only a slight amount of rash. His treatment of the disease in young persons was by venesection and cool douches. Cold water and acid drinks should be administered freely, so that sweat and other excretions may carry off poisonous materials. Care must be taken to watch the pulse, the breathing, the appearance of the feet, the evacuations from the bowels, and to modify therapy in accordance with these indications. The eruption is to be encouraged by external warmth and special care must be taken with regard to complications in the eyes, the ears, the nose, the mouth, and the pharynx.

A fact that will, perhaps, give the best idea to modern readers of the place of Rhazes in the history of medicine is that Vesalius considered it worth his while to make a translation of his principal work. Unfortunately that translation has not come down to us. When Vesalius, pestered by the controversies that had come upon him because of his venturing to make his observations for himself, accepted the post of physician to the Emperor Charles V, he burnt a number of his manuscripts. Among these were his translation of Rhazes and some annotations on Galen, which, as he says himself, had grown into a huge volume. The Galenists were bitterly decrying his refusal to accept Galen on many points, and both of these works would have added fuel to the flame of controversy. He deemed it wiser, then, not to give any further opportunities for rancorous criticism, and, feeling presumably that in his new and important post it was not worth while to bother further over the matter, he burnt them. He tells the reason in his letters to Joachin Roelant: "When I was about to leave Italy to go to Court, since a number of the physicians whom you know had made the worst kind of censure of my books, both to the Emperor himself, and to other rulers, I burned all the manuscripts that were left, although I had never suffered a moment under the displeasure of the Emperor because of these complaints, and in spite of the fact that a number of friends who were present urged me not to destroy them."

Vesalius' translation of Rhazes was probably undertaken because he recognized in him a kindred spirit of original investigation and inquiry, whose work, because it was many centuries old, would command the weight of an authority and at the same time help in the controversy over Galenic questions. This, of itself, would be quite enough to make the reputation of Rhazes, even if we did not know from the writings themselves and from the admiration of many distinguished men as well as the incentive that his works have so often proved to original observation, that he is an important link in the chain of observers in medicine, who, though we would naturally expect them to be so frequent, are really so rare.

ALI ABBAS

Rhazes lived well on into the tenth century. His successor in prestige, though not his serious rival, was Ali Ben el-Abbas, usually spoken of in medical literature as Ali Abbas, a distinguished Arabian physician who died near the end of the tenth century. He wrote a book on medicine which, because of its dedication to the Sultan, to whom he was body-physician, is known as the "Liber Regius," or "Royal Book of Medicine." This became the leading text-book of medicine for the Arabs until replaced by the "Canon of Avicenna" some two centuries later. The "Liber Regius" was an extremely practical work and, like most of the Arabian books of the early times, is simple and direct, quite without many of the objectionable features that developed later in Arabian medicine. It is valuable mainly for its contributions to diet and the fact that Ali Abbas tested many of his medicines on ailing animals before applying them to men. Of course, it owes much to earlier writers on medicine, and especially to Paul of Ægina.

An example of its practical value is to be found in his description of the treatment of a wound of the brachial artery, when, as happened often in venesection from the median basilic vein, it was injured through carelessness or inadvertence. If astringent or cauterizing methods do not stop the bleeding, the artery should be exposed, carefully isolated, tied in two places above and below the wound, and then cut across between them. He has many similar practical bits of technique. For instance, in pulling a back tooth he recommends that the gums be incised so as to loosen them around the roots, and then the tooth itself may be drawn with a special forceps which he calls a molar forceps. In ascites he recommends that when other means fail an opening should be made three finger-breadths below the navel with a pointed phlebotomy knife, and a portion of the fluid allowed to evacuate itself. A tube should then be inserted, but closed. The next day more of the fluid should be allowed to come away, and then the tube removed and the abdomen wrapped with a firm bandage.

It is easy to understand that Ali Abbas' book should have been popular, and the more we know of it the easier it is to explain why Constantine Africanus should have selected it for translation. It contains ten theoretic and ten practical books, and gives an excellent idea of the medical knowledge and medical practice of the time. Probably the fact that Constantine had translated it led to its early printing, so that we have an edition of it published at Venice in 1492, and another at Lyons in 1523. During the Middle Ages the book was often spoken of as "Regalis Dispositio," the "Royal Disposition of Medicine."

MOORISH PHYSICIANS

After Rhazes, the most important contributors to medical literature from among the Arabs, with the single exception of Avicenna, were born in Spain. They are Albucasis or

Abulcasis, the surgeon; Avenzoar, the physician, and Averroës, the philosophic theorist in medicine. Besides, it may be recalled here that Maimonides, the great Jewish physician, was born and educated at Cordova, in Spain. It might very well be a surprise that these distinguished men among the Arabs should have flourished in Spain, so far from the original seat of Arabian and Mohammedan dominion in the East, where, owing to conditions in the modern time, the English-speaking world particularly is not likely to assume that the environment was favorable for the development of science and philosophy. Anyone who recalls, however, the history of Spanish intellectual influence in the Roman Empire, as we have traced it at the beginning of this chapter, will appreciate how favorable conditions were in Spain for the fostering of intellectual development. With the disturbances that had come from political strife and the invasion of the barbarians in Italy, Spain had undoubtedly come to hold the primacy in the intellectual life of Europe at the time when the Arabs took possession of the peninsula.

ABULCASIS

The most important of the Arabian surgeons of the Middle Ages is Albucasis or Abulcasis, also Abulkasim, who was born near Cordova, in Spain. The exact year of his birth is not known, but he flourished in the second half of the tenth century. He is said to have lived to the age of 101. The name of his principal work, which embraces the whole of medicine, is "Altasrif," or "Tesrif," which has been translated "The Miscellany." Most of what he has to say about medical matters is taken from Rhazes. His work on surgery, however, in three books, represents his special contribution to the medical sciences. It contains a number of illustrations of instruments, and is the first illustrated medical book that has come to us. It was translated into Latin, and was studied very faithfully by all the surgeons of the Middle Ages. Guy de Chauliac has quoted Albucasis about two hundred times in his "Chirurgia Magna." Even as late as the beginning of the sixteenth century Fabricius de Acquapendente, the teacher of Harvey, confessed that he owed most to three great medical writers, Celsus (first century), Paul of Ægina (seventh century), and Abulcasis (tenth century).

Abulcasis insisted that for successful surgery a detailed knowledge of anatomy was, above all, necessary. He said that the reason why surgery had declined in his day was that physicians did not know their anatomy. The art of medicine, he added further, required much time. Unfortunately, to quote Hippocrates, there are many who are physicians in name only, and not in fact, especially in what regards surgery. He gives some examples of surgical mistakes made by his professional brethren that were particularly called to his attention. They are the perennially familiar instances of ignorance causing death because surgeons were tempted to operate too extensively.

His description of the procedure necessary to stop an artery from bleeding is an interesting example of his method of teaching the practical technique of surgery. Apply the finger promptly upon the opening of the vessel and press until the blood is arrested. Having heated a cautery of the appropriate size, take the finger away rapidly and touch the cautery at once to the end of the artery until the blood stops. If the spurting blood should cool the cautery, take another. There should be several ready for the purpose. Take care, he says, not to cauterize the nerves in the neighborhood, for this will add a new ailment to the patient's affection. There are only four ways of arresting arterial hemorrhage. First, by cautery; second, by division of the artery, when that is not complete—for then the extremities contract and the blood clots—or by a ligature, or by the application of substances which arrest blood flow, aided by a compressive bandage. Other means are inefficient, and seldom and, at most, accidentally successful. His instruction for first aid to the injured in case of hemorrhage in the absence of the physician, is to apply pressure directly upon the wound itself.

The development of the surgical specialties among the Arabs is particularly interesting. Abulcasis has much to say about nasal polyps. He divided them into three classes: (1) cancerous, (2) those with a number of feet, and (3) those that are soft and not living,—these latter, he says, are neither malignant nor difficult to treat. He recommends the use of a hook for their removal, or a snare for those that cannot be removed with that instrument. His instructions for the removal of objects from the external ear are interestingly practical. He advises the use of bird lime on the end of a sound to which objects will cling, or, where they are smaller, suction through a silver or copper canula. Hooks and pincettes are also suggested. Insects should be removed with a hook, or with a canula, or, having been killed by warm oil, removed by means of a syringe. Some of his observations with regard to genito-urinary surgery are quite as interesting. He even treated congenital anomalies. He suggests cutting of the meatus when narrowed, dilatation of strictures with lead sounds, and even suggests plans of operations to improve the condition in hypospadias. He gives the signs for differentiation between epitheliomata and condylomata, and distinguishes various forms of ulceration of the penis.

Abulcasis discusses varicose veins in very much the same spirit as a modern surgeon does. They occur particularly in people who work much on their feet, and especially who have to carry heavy burdens. They should not be operated on unless they produce great discomfort, and make it impossible for the sufferer to make his living. They may be operated on by means of incision or extirpation. Incision consists of cutting the veins at two or three places when they have been made prominent by means of tight bandages around the limb. The blood should be allowed to flow freely out of the cut ends, and then a bandage applied. For extirpation, the skin having been shaved beforehand, the vein should be made prominent, and then carefully laid bare. When freed from all adhesions, it should be lifted out on a hook, and either completely extirpated or several rather long pieces removed. He lays a good deal of stress on the necessity for freeing the vein thoroughly and lifting it well out of tissues before incising it. In old cases special care must be taken not to tear the vein.

Minute details of technique are often found in these old authors. Abulcasis, for instance, treats of adherent fingers with up-to-date completeness. They can occur either congenitally or from injury, as, for instance, burning. They should be separated, and then separation maintained by means of bandages or by the insertion between them of a thin lead plate, which prevents their readhesion. Adhesions of the fingers with the palm of the hand, which Abulcasis has also seen, should be treated the same way.

At times there is surprise at finding some rare lesion treated with modern technique, and a hint at least of our modern apparatus. Fracture of the pubic arch, for instance, is described in Abulcasis quite as if he had had definite experience with it. When this occurs in a woman, the reposition of the bone is often greatly facilitated by a cotton tampon in the vagina. This tampon must be removed at every urination. There is another way, however, of better securing the same purpose of counterpressure. One may take a sheep's bladder into the orifice of which a tube is fastened. One should introduce the bladder into the vagina, and then blow strongly through the tube, until the bladder becomes swollen and fills up the vaginal cavity. The fracture will, as a rule, then be readily reduced. Here is, of course, not alone the first hint of the colpeurynter, but a very practical form of the apparatus complete. Old-time physicians used the bladders of animals very generally for nearly all the medical purposes for which we now use rubber bags.

AVICENNA

Undoubtedly the most important of Abulcasis' contemporaries is the famous physician whose Arabic name, Ibn Sina, was transformed into Avicenna. He was born toward the end of the tenth century in the Persian province of Chorasan, at the height of Arabian influence, and is sometimes spoken of as the chief representative of Arabian medicine, of as much importance for it as Galen for later Greek medicine. His principal book is the so-called "Canon." It replaced the compendium "Continens" of Rhazes, and, in the East, continued until the end of the fifteenth century to be looked upon as the most complete and best system of medicine. Avicenna came to be better known in the West than any of the other Arabian writers, and his name carried great weight with it. There are very few subjects in medicine that did not receive suggestive, if not always adequate, treatment at the hands of this great Arabian medical thinker of the eleventh century. He copied freely from his predecessors, but completed their work with his own observations and conclusions. One of his chapters is devoted to leprosy alone. He has definite information with regard to bubonic plague and the *filaria medinensis*. Here and there one finds striking anticipations of what are supposed to be modern observations. Nothing was too small for his notice. One portion of the fourth book is on cosmetics, in which he treats the affections of the hair and of the nails. He has special chapters with regard to obesity, emaciation, and general constitutional conditions. His book, the "Antidotarium," is the foundation of our knowledge of the drug-giving of his time.

Some idea of the popularity and influence of Avicenna, five centuries after his time, can be readily derived from the number of commentaries on him issued during the Renaissance period by the most distinguished medical scholars and writers of that time. Hyrtl, in his "Das Arabische und Hebräische in der Anatomie," quotes some of them, — Bartholomæus de Varignana, Gentilis de Fulgineis, Jacobus de Partibus, Didacus Lopez, Jacobus de Forlivio, Ugo Senesis, Dinus de Garbo, Matthæus de Gradibus, Nicolaus Leonicenus, Thaddæus Florentinus, Galeatus de Sancta Sophia. A more complete list, with the titles of the books, may be found in Haller's "Bibliotheca Anatomica." For over three centuries after the foundation of medical schools in Europe (and even after Mondino's book had been widely distributed), Avicenna was still in the hands of all those who had an enthusiasm for medical science.

AVENZOAR

Another of the distinguished Arabian physicians was Avenzoar—the transformation of his Arabic family name, Ibn-Zohr. He was probably born in Penaflor, not far from Seville. He died in Seville in 1162 at the age, it is said, of ninety-two years. He was the son of a physician descended from a family of scholars, jurists, physicians, and officials. He received the best education of the time not only in internal medicine, but in all the specialties, and must be counted among the greatest of the Spanish Arabian physicians. He was the teacher of Averroës, who always speaks of him with great respect. He is interesting as probably being the first to suggest nutrition *per rectum*. A few words of his description show how well he knew the technique. His apparatus for the purpose consisted of the bladder of a goat or some similar animal structure,with a silver canula fastened into its neck, to be used about as we use a fountain syringe. Having first carefully washed out the rectum with cleansing and purifying clysters, he injected the nutriment—eggs, milk, and gruels—into the gut. His idea was that the intestine would take this, and, as he said, suck it up, carrying it back to the stomach, where it would be digested. He was sure that he had seen his patients benefited by it.

Some light on his studies of cases that would require such treatment may be obtained from what he has to say about the handling of a case of stricture of the esophagus. He says that this begins with some discomfort, and then some difficulty of swallowing, which is gradually and continuously increased until finally there comes complete impossibility of swallowing. It was in these cases that he suggested rectal alimentation, but he went farther than this, and treated the stricture of the esophagus itself.

The first step in this treatment is that a canula of silver or tin should be inserted through the mouth and pushed down the throat till its head meets an obstruction, always being withdrawn when there is a vomiting movement, until it becomes engaged in the stricture. Then *freshly milked* milk, or gruel made from farina or barley, should be poured through it. He says that in these cases the patient might be put in a warm milk or gruel bath, since there are some physicians who believe that through the lower parts of the body, and also through the pores of the whole body, nutrition might be taken up. While he considers that this latter method should be tried in suitable cases, he has not very much faith in it, and says that the reasons urged for it are weak and rather frivolous. It is easy to understand that a man who has reached the place in medicine where he can recommend manipulative treatments of this kind, and discuss nutritional modes so rationally, knew his practical medicine well, and wrote of it judiciously.

AVERROËS

Among the distinguished contributors to medicine at this time, though more a philosopher than a physician, is the famous Averroës, whose full Arabic name among his contemporaries was Abul-Welid Mohammed Ben Ahmed Ibn Roschd el-Maliki. Like Avenzoar, of whom he was the intimate personal friend, and Abulcasis and Maimonides, he was born in the south of Spain. He was in high favor with the King of Morocco and of Spain, El-Mansur Jacub, often known as Almansor, who made him one of his counsellors. His works are much more important for philosophy than for medicine, and his philosophical writings gave him a place only second to that of Aristotle in the Western world during the Middle Ages. Averroism is still a subject of at least academic interest, and Renan's monograph on it and its author was one of the popular books of the latter half of the nineteenth century in philosophic circles. In spite of his friendship with the Moorish King and with Avenzoar, he fell under the suspicion of free thinking and was brought to trial with a number of personal friends, who occupied high positions in the Moorish government. He escaped with his life, but only after great risks, and he was banished to a suburb of Cordova, in which only Jews were allowed to live. By personal influence he succeeded in securing the pardon of himself and friends, and then was summoned to the court of the son and successor of El-Mansur in Morocco. He died, not long after, in 1198.

Altogether there are some thirty-three works of Averroës on philosophy and science. Only three of these are concerned with medicine. One is the "Colliget," so-called, containing seven books, on anatomy, physiology, pathology, diagnostics, materia medica, hygiene, and therapy. Then there is a commentary on the "Cantica of Avicenna," and a tractate on the "Theriac." Averroës' idea in writing about medicine was to apply his particular system of philosophy to medical science. His intimate relations with other great physicians of the time, and in particular his close friendship with Avenzoar, enabled him to get abundant medical information in faultless order so far as knowledge then went, but his theoretic speculations, instead of helping medicine, as he thought they would, and as philosophers have always been inclined to think as regards their theoretic contributions, were not only not of value, but to some extent at least hindered human progress by diverting men from the field of observation to that of speculation. It is interesting to realize that Averroës did in his time what Descartes did many centuries later, and many another brilliant thinker has done before and since.

ARABIAN INFLUENCE

The fame of these great thinkers and writers in philosophy and in medicine came to be known not only through the distribution of their books long after their death, but during their lifetime, and in immediately subsequent generations, ardent seekers after knowledge, who were themselves afterwards to become famous by their teaching and writing, found their way into the Arabian dominions in order to take advantage of the educational opportunities afforded. These were better than they could secure at home in Christian countries, because the process of bringing culture and devotion to literature and science into the minds of the Northern nations, who had replaced the old Romans in Europe, was not yet completed. Bagdad and Cordova were the two favorite places of educational pilgrimage. The names that are most familiar among the scholars in the Middle Ages in Europe are those of whom it is recorded that they made long journeys in order to get in touch with what the Arabs had preserved of the old Greek civilization and culture. Among them are such men as Michael Scot or Scotus, Matthew Platearius, who was afterwards a great teacher at Salerno; Daniel Morley, Adelard of Bath, Egidius, otherwise known as Gilles de Corbeil; Romoaldus, Gerbert of Auvergne, who later became Pope under the name of Sylvester II; Gerard of Cremona, and the best known of them all, at least in medicine, Constantine Africanus, whose wanderings, however, were probably not limited to Arabian lands, but who seems also to have been in Hindustan.

We are rather prone to think that this great spirit of going far afield for knowledge's sake is recent, or, at least, quite modern. As a matter of fact, one finds it everywhere in history. Long before Herodotus did his wanderings there were many visitors who went to Egypt, and many more later who went to Crete, and many more a few centuries later who went to the shores of Asia Minor seeking for the precious pearl of knowledge, and sometimes finding it without finding the even more precious pearl of wisdom, "whose worth is from the farthest coasts."

To the Arabs we owe the foundation of a series of institutions for the higher learning, like those which had existed around them in Asia Minor and in Egypt at the time they made their conquests. Alexandria, Pergamos, Cos, Cnidos, Tarsus, and many other Eastern cities had had what we would call at least academies, and many of them deserved the name of universities. The Arabs continued the tradition in education that they found, and established educational institutions which attracted wide attention. As we have said, the two most famous of these were at Bagdad and at Cordova. Mostanser, the predecessor of the last Caliph of the family of the Abbassides, built a handsome palace, in which the academy of Bagdad was housed. It is still in existence, and gives an excellent idea of the beneficent interest of this monarch and of other of the Abbasside rulers in education. Its fate at the present time is typical of the attitude of the Mohammed ans towards education. Though the building is still standing, the institution of learning is no longer there. As Hyrtl remarks, it is not ideas that are exchanged in it now, but articles of commerce. It has become the chief office of the Turkish customs department in Bagdad.

These institutions of the higher learning, founded by the Arabs, at first as rather strict imitations of the museums or academies of Egypt and Asia Minor, gradually changed their character under the Arabs. Their courses became much more formal, examinations became much more important. Scholarship was sought not so much for its own sake, as because it led to positions in the civil service, to the favor of princes, and, in general, to reputation and pecuniary reward. Formal testimonials proclaiming education, signed by the academic authorities, were introduced and came to mean much. Lawyers could not practise without a license, physicians also required a license. These formalities were adopted by the Western medieval universities to a considerable degree and have been perpetuated in the modern time. Undoubtedly they did much to hamper real education among the Arabs by setting in place of the satisfaction of learning for its own sake and the commendation of teachers the formal recognition of a certain amount of work done as recognized by the educational authorities. There was always a tendency among the Arabs to formulate and formalize, to over-systematize what they were at; to think that new knowledge could be obtained simply by speculating over what was already acquired, and developing it. There are a number of comparisons between this and later periods of education that might be suggested if comparisons were not odious.

The influence of Arabian medicine on modern medicine can, perhaps, best be judged from the number of words in our modern nomenclature, which, though bearing Latin forms, often with suggestion of Greek origins, still are not derived from the old Latin or Greek authors, but represent Arabic terms translated into Latin during the Renaissance period. Hyrtl, without pretence of quoting them all, gives a list of these which is surprising in its comprehensiveness. For instance, the mediastinum, the sutura sagittalis, the scrobiculus cordis, the marsupium cordis, the chambers of the heart, the velum palati, the trochanter, the rima glottidis, the fontanelles, the alæ of the nose, all have their present names, not from original Latin expressions, but from the translation of Arabic terms. For all such words the Greeks and Romans have quite other expressions, in which the sense of our modern terms is not contained. This has given rise to many misunderstandings, and to many attempts in the modern times to return to the classic terminology rather than preserve what in many cases are the barbarisms introduced through the Arabic, but it is doubtful whether any comprehensive reform in the matter can be effected, so strongly entrenched in medical usage have these terms now become.

Freind, in his "History of Medicine," already cited, calls attention to the fact that the Arabs had an unfortunate tendency to change by addition or subtraction of their own views the authors that they studied, and wished to translate to others. This seems to have been true even of some of the most distinguished of them. Of course, the idea of preserving an author's text untouched, and making it clear just where note and commentary came in, had not yet come to men's view, but quite apart from this the Arabs apparently often tried to gain acceptance for their own ideas by having them masquerade as the supposed ideas of favorite classic authors.

Another unfortunate tendency among the Arabs was their liking for the discussion of many trivial questions. Hyrtl, in his volume on "Arabian and Hebrew Words in Anatomy,"[6] declares that it is almost incredible how earnestly some trivial questions in anatomy and physiology were discussed by the Arabs. He gives some examples. Why does no hair grow on the nose of men? Why does the stomach not lie behind the mouth? Why does the windpipe not lie behind the esophagus? Why are the breasts not on the abdomen? Why are not the calves on the anterior portion of the legs? Even such men as Rhazes and Avicenna discuss such questions.

It was this tendency of the Arabs that passed over to the Western Europeans with Arabian commentaries on philosophy and science, and brought so many similar discussions in the scholastic period. These trivialities have usually been supposed to originate with the scholastics themselves, for they are not to be found in the Greek authors on whom the scholastics were writing commentaries, but they are typically Oriental in character, and it must be remembered that during the twelfth and early thirteenth centuries, at least, Greek philosophy found its way largely into Europe in Arab versions, and these characteristically Arabian additions of the discussion of curious trivial questions came with them and produced an imitative tendency among the Europeans.

As a rule the more careful has been the study of Arabian writers in the modern time, particularly by specialists, the clearer has it become that they lacked nearly all originality. Especially were they faulty in their observations; besides, they had a definite tendency to replace observation by theory, a fatal defect in medicine. The fine development of surgery that came at the end of the Arabian period of medicine in Europe could never have come from the Arabs themselves. Gurlt has brought this out particularly, but it will not be difficult to cite many other good authorities in support of this opinion.

Hyrtl, in his "Thesis on the Rarer Old Anatomists,"[7] says that "the Arabs paid very little attention to anatomy, and, of course, because of the prohibition in the Koran, added nothing to it. Whatever they knew they took from the Greeks, and especially Galen. Not only did they not add anything new to this, but they even lost sight of much that was important in the older authors. The Arabs were much more interested in physiology; they could study this by giving thought to it without soiling their hands. They delighted in theory, rather than in observation."

While we thus discuss the lack of originality and the tendency to over-refinement among the Arabian medical writers, it must not be thought that we would make little of what they accomplished. They not only preserved the old medical writers for us, but they kept alive practical medicine with the principles of the great Greek thinkers as its basis. There are a large number of writers of Arabian medicine whose names have secured deservedly a high place in medical history. If this were a formal history of Arabian medicine, their careers and works would require discussion. For our purpose, however, it seems better to confine attention to a few of the most prominent Arabian writers on medicine, because they will serve to illustrate how thoroughly practical were the Arabian physicians and how many medical problems that we are prone to think of as modern they occupied themselves with, solving them not infrequently nearly as we do in the modern time.

VI

THE MEDICAL SCHOOL AT SALERNO

The Medical School at Salerno, probably organized early in the tenth century, often spoken of as the darkest of the centuries, and reaching its highest point of influence at the end of the twelfth century, is of great interest in modern times for a number of reasons. First it brought about in the course of its development an organization of medical education, and an establishment of standards that were to be maintained whenever and wherever there was a true professional spirit down to our own time. They insisted on a preliminary education of three years of college work, on at least four years of medical training, on special study for specialist's work, as in surgery, and on practical training with a physician or in a hospital before the student was allowed to practise for himself. At Salerno, too, the department of women's diseases was given over to women professors, and we have the text-books of some of these women medical teachers. The license to practise given to women, however, seems to have been general and did not confine them merely to the care of women and children. We have records of a number of these licenses issued to women in the neighborhood of Salerno. This subject of feminine medical education at Salerno, because of its special interest in our time, will have a chapter by itself.

These are the special features of medical education in our own time that we are rather prone to think of as originating with ourselves and as being indices of that evolution of humanity and progress in mankind which are culminating in our era. It is rather interesting, then, to study just how these developments came about and what the genesis of this great school was. The books of its professors were widely read, not only in their own generation but for centuries afterwards. With the invention of printing at the time of the Renaissance most of them were printed and exerted profound influence over the revival of medicine which took place at that time. Salerno became the first of the universities in the modern sense of the word. Here there gathered round the medical school, first a preparatory department representing modern college work, and then departments of theology and law, though this latter department particularly was never quite successful. The fact that the first university, that of Salerno, should have been organized round a medical school, the second, that of Bologna, around a law school, and the third, that of Paris, around a school of theology and philosophy, would seem to represent the ordinary natural process of development in human interests. First man is interested in himself and in his health, then in his property, and finally in his relations to his fellow-man and to God.

Though much work has been done on the subject in recent years, it is not easy to trace the origin of the medical school at Salerno. The difficulty is emphasized by the fact that even the earliest chroniclers whose accounts we have were not sure as to its origin, and even had some doubt about the age of the school. Alphanus, usually designated Alphanus I because there are several of the name, who is one of the earliest professors whose name and fame have come down to us, gives us the only definite detail as to the age of the school. He was a Benedictine monk, distinguished as a literary man, known both as poet and physician, who was afterwards raised to the Bishopric of Salerno. As a bishop he was one of the beneficent patrons, to whom the school owed much. He lived in the tenth century, and states that medicine flourished in the town before the time of Guimarus II, who reigned in the ninth century. In the ancient chronicle of Salerno, re-discovered by De Renzi and published in his "Collectio Salernitana," it is definitely recorded that the medical school was founded by four doctors,—a Jewish Rabbi Elinus, a Greek Pontus, a Saracen Adala, an Arab, and a native of Salerno, each of whom lectured in his native language. There are many elements in this tradition, however, that would seem to indicate its mythical origin and that it was probably invented after the event to account for the presence of teachers in all these languages and the coming of students from all over the world. The names, for instance, are apparently corruptions of real names, as can be readily recognized. Elinus, the Jew, is probably Elias or Eliseus, Adala is a corruption of Abdallah, and Pontus, as pointed out by Puschmann in his "History of Medical Education," should probably be Gario-Pontus.

While we do not know exactly when the medical school at Salerno was founded, we know that a hospital was established there as early as 820. It was founded by the Archdeacon Adelmus, and was placed under the control of the Benedictines after it was realized that a religious order, by its organization, was best fitted for carrying on such charitable work continuously. Other infirmaries and charitable institutions, mainly under control of the religious, sprang up in Salerno. It was the presence of these hospitals in a salubrious climate that seems first to have attracted the attention of patients and then of physicians from all over Europe and even adjacent Africa and Asia. Puschmann says that it is uncertain whether clinical instruction was imparted in these institutions or not, but the whole tenor of what we know about the practical character of the teaching at Salerno and of the fine development of professional medicine there, would seem to argue that probably those who came to study medicine here were brought directly in contact with patients.

As early as the ninth century Salerno was famous for its great physicians. We know the names of at least two physicians, Joseph and Joshua, who practised there about the middle of the ninth century. Ragenifrid, a Lombard by his name, was private physician to Prince Wyamar of Salerno in the year 900. The fact that he was from North Italy indicates that already foreigners were being attracted, but more than this that they were obtaining opportunities unhampered by any Chauvinism. From early in the tenth century physicians from Salerno were frequently brought to foreign courts to become the attending physicians to rulers. Patients of the highest distinction from all over Europe began to flock to Salerno, and we have the names of many of them. In the tenth century Bishop Adalberon, when ailing, went there, though he found no cure for his ills. Abbot Desiderius, however, the great Benedictine scholar of the time, who afterwards became Pope Victor

III, regained his health at Salerno under the care of the great Constantine Africanus, who was so much impressed by the gentle kindness and deep learning and the example of the saintly life of his patient that not long after he went to Monte Cassino to become a Benedictine under Desiderius, who was abbot there. Duke Guiscard sent his son Bohemund to Salerno for the cure of a wound received in battle, which had refused to heal under the ordinary surgical treatment of the time. William the Conqueror, early in the eleventh century and while still only the Duke of Normandy, is said to have passed some time at Salerno for a similar reason.

The most interesting feature of the medical life at Salerno at this time is the relations between the clergy and the physicians. In the sketch of the life of Constantine Africanus, which follows this chapter, there is some account of the friendship between Abbot Desiderius of Monte Cassino and Constantine Africanus, and the latter's withdrawal from his professorship to become a Benedictine. One of the physicians of the early tenth century who stood high in favor with Prince Gisulf was raised to the Bishopric of Salerno. This was Alphanus, whom we have already mentioned as a chronicler, a monk, a poet, a physician, and finally the Bishop of Salerno.

The best proof of how thorough was the medical education at Salerno and how much influence it exerted even over public opinion is to be found in the regulation of the practice of medicine, which soon began, and the insistence upon proper training before permission to practise medicine was granted. The medical school at Salerno early came to be a recognized institution in the kingdom of the Two Sicilies, representing a definite standard of medical training. It is easy to understand that the attraction which Salerno possessed for patients soon also brought to the neighborhood a number of irregular physicians, travelling quacks, and charlatans. Wealthy patients were coming from all over the world to be treated at Salerno. Many of them doubtless were sufferers from incurable diseases and nothing could be done for them. Often they would be quite unable to return to their homes and would be surely unwilling to give up all hope if anybody promised them anything of relief. There was a rich field for the irregular, and of course, as always, he came. Salerno had already shown what a good standard of medical education should be, and it is not surprising, then, that the legal authorities in this part of the country proceeded to the enforcement of legal regulations demanding the attainment of this standard, in order that unfit and unworthy physicians might not practise medicine to their own benefit but to the detriment of the patients.

Accordingly, as early as the year 1140, King Ruggiero (Roger) of the Two Sicilies promulgated the law: "Whoever from this time forth desires to practise medicine must present himself before our officials and judges, and be subject to their decision.Anyone audacious enough to neglect this shall be punished by imprisonment and confiscation of goods. This decree has for its object the protection of the subjects of our kingdom from the dangers arising from the ignorance of practitioners."

Just about a century later the Emperor Frederick II, the Hohenstaufen, in the year 1240, extended this law, emphasized it, and brought it particularly into connection with the great medical school of the Two Sicilies, of which territory he was the ruler. This law has often been proclaimed as due to his personality rather than to his times,—as representing his very modern spirit and his progressive way of looking at things. There is no doubt that certain personal elements for which he should be given due credit are contained in the law. To understand it properly, however, one must know the law of King Roger of the preceding century; and then it is easy to appreciate that Frederick's regulation is only such a development of the governmental attitude toward medical practice as might have been expected during the century since Roger's time. It has sometimes been suggested that this law made by the Emperor Frederick, who was so constantly in bitter opposition to the Papacy, was issued in despite of the Church authorities and represents a policy very different from any which they would have encouraged. The early history of Salerno, even briefly as we have given it, completely contradicts any such idea. The history of medical regulation at the beginning of the next century down at Montpellier moreover, where the civil authorities being weak the legal ordering of the practice of medicine was effectively taken up by the Church, and the authority for the issuance of licenses to practise was in the hands of the bishops of the neighborhood, shows clearly that it is not because of any knowledge of the real medical history of the times that such remarks are made, but from a set purpose to discredit the Church.

The Emperor Frederick's law deserves profound respect and consideration because of the place that it holds in the legal regulation of the practice of medicine. Anyone who thinks that evolution must have brought us in seven centuries much farther in this matter than were the people of the later Middle Ages should read this law attentively. Everyone who is interested in medical education should have a copy of it near him, because it will have a chastening effect in demonstrating not only how little we have done in the modern time rather than how much, but above all how much of decadence there was during many periods of the interval. The law may be found in the original in "The Popes and Science" (Fordham University Press, N. Y., 1908). Three years of preliminary university education before the study of medicine might be taken up, four years of medical studies proper before a degree was given, a year of practice with a regularly licensed physician before a license to practise could be obtained, a special course in anatomy if surgery were to be practised; all this represents an ideal we are striving after at the present time in medical education. Besides this, Frederick's law also regulates medical fees, requires gratuitous attendance on the poor for the privilege of practice accorded by the license, though the general fees are of a thoroughly professional character and represent for each visit of the physician about the amount of daily wage that the ordinary laborer of that time earned. Curiously enough, this same ratio of emolument has maintained itself. This law was also a pure drug law, regulating the practice of pharmacy, and the price as well as the purity of drugs, and the relations of physicians, druggists, and the royal drug inspectors whose business it was to see that only proper drugs were prepared and sold.

All this is so much more advanced than we could possibly have imagined, only that the actual documents are in our possession, that most people refuse to let themselves be persuaded in spite of the law that it could have meant very much. Especially as regards medical education are they dubious as to conditions at this time. To them it seems that it can make very little difference how much time was required for medical study or for studies preliminary to medicine, since there was so little to be learned. The age was ignorant, men knew but little, and so very little could be imparted no matter how much time was taken.

This is, I fear, a common impression, but an utterly false one. The preliminary training that is the undergraduate work at the universities consisted of the Seven Liberal Arts

—the trivium and quadrivium, which embraced logic, rhetoric, grammar, metaphysics, under which was included not a little of physics, cosmology in which some biology was studied, as well as psychology and mathematics, astronomy, and music. This was a thoroughly rounded course in intellectual training. No wonder that Professor Huxley said in his Inaugural Address as Rector of Aberdeen, "I doubt if the curriculum of any modern university shows so clear and generous a comprehension of what is meant by culture as this old trivium and quadrivium does." There is no doubt at all about the value of the undergraduate training, nor of the scholarship of the men who were turned out under the system, nor of their ability to concentrate their minds on difficult subjects—a faculty that we strive to cultivate in our time and do not always congratulate ourselves on securing to the degree, at least, that we would like.

As to the medical teaching, Ægidius, often called Gilles of Corbeil, who was a graduate of Salerno and afterward became the physician-in-ordinary to Philip Augustus, King of France, thought that he could not say too much for the training in medicine that was given at this first of the medical schools. One thing is sure, the professors were eminently serious, the work taken up was in many ways thoroughly scientific, and some of the results of the medical investigations of that early day are interesting even now. The descriptions of diseases that we have from the Salernitan school are true to nature and are replete with many original observations. Puschmann says: "The accounts given of intermittent fever, pneumonia, phthisis, psoriasis, lupus, which they called the malum mortuum, of ulcers on the sexual organs, among which it is easy to recognize chancre, and of the disturbances of the mental faculties, especially deserve mention." They seem to have been quite expert in their knowledge of phthisis. In the treatment of it they laid great stress upon the giving up of a strenuous life, the living a rather easy existence in the open air, and a suitable diet. When the commencement of consumption was suspected, the first prescription was a good course of strengthening nourishment for the patient. On the other hand, they declared that the cases in which diarrhea supervened during consumption soon proved fatal. In general, with regard to people who were liable to respiratory diseases, they insisted upon life in an atmosphere of equable temperature. Though the custom was almost unheard of in the Salerno of that time, and indeed at the present time there is very little heating during the winter in southern Italy, they insisted that patients who were liable to pulmonary affections should have their rooms heated.

On the other hand, they suggested the cooling of the air of the sick-room, as we have noted in the chapter on Constantine Africanus, and Afflacius recommended the employment of an apparatus from which water trickled continuously in drops to the ground and then evaporated. Baths and bleeding were employed according to definite indications and diet was always a special feature. They had a number of drugs and simples, and the employment of some of them is interesting. Iron was prescribed for enlargement of the spleen. The internal use of sea sponge, in which of course there is a noteworthy proportion of iodine, was recommended for relief from the symptoms of goitre by reducing its size. Iodine has been used so much ever since in this affection, even down to our own day, that this employment of one of its compounds is rather striking.Massage of the goitre was also recommended, and this mode of treatment was commonly employed for a number of ailments.

Probably the best idea that can be obtained in brief space of the achievements of the University of Salerno is to be found in Pagel's appreciation of Salerno's place in the history of medicine in his chapters on "Medicine in the Middle Ages" in Puschmann's "Handbuch der Geschichte der Medizin" (Berlin, 1902). He said: "If we take up now the accomplishments of the school of Salerno in the different departments there is one thing that is very remarkable. It is the rich independent productivity with which Salerno advanced the banners of medical science for hundreds of years almost as the only autochthonous centre of medical influence in the whole West. One might almost say that it was like a *versprengten Keim*—a displaced embryonic element—which, as it unfolded, rescued from destruction the ruined remains of Greek and Roman medicine. This productivity of Salerno, which may well be compared in quality and quantity with that of the best periods of our science, and in which no department of medicine was left without some advance, is one of the striking phenomena of the history of medicine. While positive progress was not made, there are many noteworthy original observations to be chronicled. It must be acknowledged that pupils and scholars set themselves faithfully to their tasks to further as far as their strength allowed the science and art of healing. In the medical writers of the older period of Salerno who had not yet been disturbed by Arabian culture or scholasticism, we cannot but admire the clear, charmingly smooth, light-flowing diction, the delicate and honest setting forth of cases, the simplicity of their method of treatment, which was to a great extent dietetic and expectant, and while we admire the carefulness and yet the copiousness of their therapy, we cannot but envy them a certain austerity in their pharmaceutic formulas and an avoidance of medicamental polypragmasia. The work in internal medicine was especially developed. The contributions to it from a theoretic and a literary standpoint, as well as from practical applications, found ardent devotees."

Less than this could scarcely have been expected from the medical school which brought such an uplift of professional dignity and advance in the standards of medical education that are to be noticed in connection with Salerno. Registration, licensure, preliminary education, adequate professional studies, clinical experience under expert guidance, even special training for surgical work, all came in connection with this great medical school. Such practical progress in medical education could not have been made but by men who faced the problems of the practice of medicine without self-deception and solved them as far as possible by common-sense, natural, and rational methods.

It is usually said that at Salerno surgery occupied an inferior position. It is true that we have less record of it in the earlier years of Salerno than we would like to see. It was somewhat handicapped by the absence of human dissection. This very important defect was not due to any Church opposition to anatomy, as has often been said, but to the objection that people have to seeing the bodies of their friends or acquaintances used for anatomical purposes. In the comparatively small towns of the Middle Ages there were few strangers, and therefore very seldom were there unclaimed bodies. The difficulty was in the obtaining of dissecting material. We had the same difficulty in this country until about two generations ago, and the only way that bodies could be obtained regularly was by "resurrecting" them, as it was called, from graveyards. In the absence of human subjects, anatomy was taught at Salerno upon the pig. The principal portion of the teaching in anatomy consisted of the demonstration of the organs in the great cavities of the body and their relations, with some investigations of their form and the presumed functions of the corresponding organs in man.

Copho's well-known "Anatomy of the Pig" was a text-book written for the students of Salerno. In spite of its limitations, it shows the beginnings of rather searching original inquiry and even some observations in pathological anatomy. It is simple and straightforward and does not profess to be other than it is, though it must be set down as the first reasonably complete contribution to comparative anatomy.

When their surgery came to be written down, however, it gave abundant evidence of the thoroughness with which this department of medicine had been cultivated by the Salernitan faculty. We have the text-book of Roger, with the commentary of Rolando, and then the so-called commentary of the Four Masters. These writings were probably made rather for the medical school at Bologna than that of Salerno, though there is no doubt that at least Roger and Rolando received their education at Salerno and embodied in their writings the surgical traditions of that school. While I have preferred, in order to have a connected story of surgical development, to treat of their contributions to their specialty under the head of the "Great Surgeons of the Medieval Universities," it seems well to point out here that they must be considered as representing especially the surgical teaching of the older medical school of Salerno. There are many interesting features of the old teaching that they have embodied in their books. For instance, at Salerno both sutures and ligatures were employed in order to prevent bleeding. We are rather accustomed to think of such uses of thread, and especially the ligature, as being much later inventions. The fact of the matter is, however, that ligatures and sutures were reinvented over and over again and then allowed to go out of use until someone who had no idea of their dangers came to reinvent them once more.[8]

Much is often said about the place of Arabian surgery and medicine at this time, and the influence that they had over the medical teaching and thinking of the period. To trust many of the shorter histories of medicine the Arabs must be given credit for more of the medical thought of this time than any other medical writers or thinkers. It is forgotten, however, apparently, that in the southern part of Italy, where Salerno was situated, Greek influence never died out. This had been a Greek colony in the olden time and continued to be known for many centuries after the Christian era as Magna Græcia. Greek medicine, then, had more influence here than anywhere else. As a matter of fact, the beginnings of Salernitan teaching are all Greek and not at all Arabian. This is as true in surgery as in medicine. I have quoted Gurlt in the chapter on "Great Surgeons of the Medieval Universities," insisting that the Salernitan school owed nothing at all to Arabian surgery. Salernitan medicine was, during the twelfth century, just as free from Arabian influence. When Arabian medicine makes itself felt, as pointed out by Pagel in his "Geschichte der Heilkunde im Mittelalter,"[9] far from exerting a beneficial influence, it had a rather unfortunate effect. It led especially to an oversophistication of medicine from the standpoint of drug therapeutics. The Arabian physicians trusted nature very little. In this they were like our forefathers of medicine one hundred years ago, of whom Rush was the typical representative—so history repeats itself.

Before the introduction of Arabian medicine the Salernitan school of medicine was noted for its common-sense methods and its devotion to all the natural modes of healing. It looked quite as much to the prevention of disease as its treatment. Diet and air and water were always looked upon as significant therapeutic aids. With the coming of Arabian influence there began, says Pagel, "as the literature of the times shows very well, that rule of the apothecary in therapeutics which was an unfortunate exaggeration. Now all the above-mentioned complicated prescriptions came to be the order of the day. Apparently the more complicated a prescription the better. Dietetics especially was relegated to the background. Salerno, at the end of the twelfth century, had already reached its highest point of advance in medicine and was beginning to decline. Decadence was evident in so far as all the medical works that we have from that time are either borrowings or imitations from Arabian medicine with which eventually Salernitan medical literature became confounded. Only a few independent authors are found after this time." This is so very different from what is ordinarily presumed to have been the case and openly proclaimed by many historians of medicine because apparently they would prefer to attribute scientific advance to the Arabs than to the Christian scholars of the time, that it is worth while noting it particularly.

Salerno was particularly rich in its medical literary products. Very often we have not the names of the writers. Apparently there is good reason to think that a number of the professors consulted together in writing a book, and when it was issued it was considered to be a text-book of the Salernitan school of medicine rather than of any particular professor. This represents a development of co-operation on the part of colleagues in medical teaching that we are likely to think of as reserved for much later times.

The most important medical writing that comes to us from Salerno, in the sense at least of the work that has had most effect on succeeding generations, has been most frequently transcribed, most often translated and committed to memory by many generations of physicians, is the celebrated Salernitan medical poem on hygiene. The title of the original Latin was "Regimen Sanitatis Salernitanum." It was probably written about the beginning of the twelfth century. A century or so later it came to be the custom to call medical books after flowers, and so we had the "Lilium Medicinæ" and the "Flos Medicinæ" down at Montpellier, and this became the "Flos

Medicinæ" of Salerno. Pagel calls it the quintessence of Salernitan therapeutics.

For many centuries portions at least of this Latin medical poem were as common in the mouths of physicians all over Europe as the aphorisms of Hippocrates or the sayings of Galen. Probably this enables us to understand the great reputation that the Salernitan school enjoyed and the influence that it wielded better than anything else. The poem is divided into ten principal parts, containing altogether about 3,500 lines. The first part on hygiene has 855 lines in eight chapters. The second part on *materia medica*, though containing only four chapters, has also about 800 lines. Anatomy and physiology are crowded into about 200 lines, etiology has something over 200, semiotics has about 250, pathology has but thirty lines more or less, and therapeutics about 400; nosology has about 600 more, and finally there is something about the physician himself, and an epilogue. As Latin verses go, when written for such purposes, these are not so bad, though some of them would grate on a literary ear. The whole work makes a rather interesting compendium of medicine, with therapeutic indications and contra-indications, and whatever the physician of the medieval period needed to have ready to memory. Some of its prescriptions, both in the sense of formulæ and of directions to the patient, have quite a modern air.

One very interesting contribution to medical literature that comes to us from Salerno bears the title, "The Coming of a Physician to His Patient, or An Instruction for the Physician Himself." We have had a number of such works published in recent years, but it is a little surprising to have the subject taken up thus early in the history of modern professional life. It is an extremely valuable document, as demonstrating how practical was the teaching at Salerno. The work is usually ascribed to Archimattheas, and it certainly gives a vivid picture of the medical customs of the time. The instruction for the immediate coming of the physician to his patient runs as follows: "When the doctor enters the dwelling of his patient, he should not appear haughty, nor covetous, but should greet with kindly, modest demeanor those who are present, and then seating himself near the sick man accept the drink which is offered him (*sic*) and praise in a few words the beauty of the neighborhood, the situation of the house, and the well-known generosity of the family,—if it should seem to him suitable to do so. The patient should be put at his ease before the examination begins and the pulse should be felt deliberately and carefully. The fingers should be kept on the pulse at least until the hundredth beat in order to judge its kind and character; the friends standing round will be all the more impressed because of the delay and the physician's words will be received with just that much more attention."

The old physician evidently realized very well how much influence on the patient's mind meant for the course of the disease. For instance, he recommends that the patient should be asked to confess and receive the sacraments of the Church before the doctor sees him, for if mention is afterwards made of this the patient may believe that it is because the doctor thinks that there is no hope for him. For the purpose of producing an effect upon the patient's mind, the old physician does not hesitate even to suggest the taking advantage of every possible source of information, so as to seem to know all about the case. "On the way to see the sick person he [the physician] should question the messenger who has summoned him upon the circumstances and the conditions of the illness of the patient; then, if not able to make any positive diagnosis after examining the pulse and the urine, he will at least excite the patient's astonishment by his accurate knowledge of the symptoms of the disease and thus win his confidence."

At the end of these preliminary instructions there is a rather diplomatic—to say the least—bit of advice that might perhaps to a puritanic conscience seem more politic than truthful. Since the old professor insists so much on not disturbing the patient's mind by a bad prognosis or any hint of it, and since even some exaggeration of what he might think to be the serious outlook of the case to friends would only lead to greater care of the patient, there is probably much more justification for his suggestion than might be thought at first glance. He says, "When the doctor quits the patient he should promise him that he will get quite well again, but he should inform his friends that he is very ill; in this way, if a cure is affected, the fame of the doctor will be so much the greater, but if the patient dies people will say that the doctor had foreseen the fatal issue."

The story of the medical school of Salerno, even thus briefly and fragmentarily told, illustrates very well how old is the new in education,—even in medical education. There is scarcely a phase of modern interest in medical education that may not be traced very clearly at Salerno though the school began its career a thousand years ago, and ceased to attract much attention over six hundred years ago. We owe most of our knowledge of the details of its organization and teaching to De Renzi. Without the devotion of so ardent a scholar it would have been almost impossible for us to have attained so complete a picture of Salernitan activities. As it is, as a consequence of his work we are able to see this first of modern medical schools developing very much as do our most modern medical schools. There has been an accumulation of medical information in the thousand years, but the ways and modes of facing problems and many of the solutions of them do not differ from what they were in the distant past. The more we know about any particular period, the more is this brought home to us. It is for this that study of particular periods and institutions of the olden time, as of

Salerno, grows increasingly interesting, because each new detail helps to fill in sympathetically the new-old picture of human activity as it may be seen at all times.

VII

CONSTANTINE AFRICANUS

Probably the most important representative of the medical school at Salerno, certainly the most significant member of its faculty, if we consider the wide influence for centuries after his time that his writings had, was Constantine Africanus. He is interesting, too, for many other reasons, for he is the first representative, in modern times, that is, who, after the incentive of antiquity had passed, devoted himself to creating a medical literature by translations, by editions, and by the collation of his own and others' observations on medical subjects. He is the connecting link between Arabian medicine and Western medical studies. The fact that he was first a traveller over most of the educational world of his time, then a professor at the University of Salerno who attracted many students, and finally a Benedictine monk in the great abbey at Monte Cassino, shows how his life ran the gamut of the various phases of interest in the intellectual world of his time. It was his retirement to the famous monastery that gave him the opportunity, the leisure, the reference library for consultation that a writer feels he must have near him, and probably also the means necessary for the publication of his works. Not only did the monks of Monte Cassino itself de vote themselves to the copying of his many books, but other Benedictine monasteries in various parts of the world made it a point to give wide diffusion to his writings.

As a study in successful publication, that is, in the securing of wide attention to writings within a short time, the career of Constantine and the story of his books would be extremely interesting. Medieval distribution of books is usually thought to have been rather halting, but here was an exception. It was largely because Benedictines all over the world were deeply interested in what this brother Benedictine was writing that wide distribution was secured for his work within a very short time. His superiors among the Benedictines had a profound interest in what he was doing. The great Benedictine Abbot Desiderius of Monte Cassino, who afterwards became Pope, used all of his extensive influence in both positions to secure an audience for the books—hence the many manuscript copies of his writings that we have. It is probable that Constantine established a school of writers at Monte Cassino, for he could scarcely have accomplished so much by himself as has been attributed to him. Besides, his works attracted so much attention that writers of immediately succeeding generations who wanted to secure attention for their works sometimes attributed them to him in order to take advantage of his popularity. It is rather difficult, then, to determine with absolute assurance which are Constantine's genuine works. Some of those attributed to him are undoubtedly spurious. What we know with certainty, however, is that his authentic works meant much for his own and after generations.

Constantine was born in the early part of the eleventh century, and died near its close, having lived probably well beyond eighty years of age, his years running nearly parallel with his century. His surname, Africanus, is derived from his having been born in Africa, his birthplace being Carthage. Early in life he seems to have taken up with ardor the study of medicine in his native town, devoting himself, however, at the same time to whatever of physical science was available. Like many another young man since his time, not satisfied with the knowledge he could secure at home, he made distant journeys, gathering medical and scientific information of all kinds wherever he went. According to a tradition that seems to be well grounded, some of these journeys took him even into the far East. During his travels he became familiar with a number of Oriental languages, and especially studied the Arabian literature of science very diligently.

At this time the Arabs, having the advantage of more intimate contact with the Greek medical traditions in Asia Minor, were farther advanced in their knowledge of the medical sciences than the scholars in the West. They had better facilities for obtaining the books that were the classics of medicine, and, with any desire for knowledge, could scarcely fail to secure it.

What was best in Arabian medicine was brought to Salerno by Constantine and, above all, his translation of many well-known Arabian medical authors proved eminently suggestive to seriously investigating physicians all over the world in his time. Before he was to be allowed to settle down to his literary work, however, Constantine was to have a very varied experience. Some of this doubtless was to be valuable in enabling him to set the old Arabian teachers of medicine properly before his generation. After his Oriental travels he returned to his native Carthage in order to practise medicine. It was not long, however, before his superior medical knowledge, or, at least, the many novelties of medical practice that he had derived from his contact with the East, drew upon him the professional jealousy of his colleagues. It is very probable that the reputation of his extensive travels and wide knowledge soon attracted a large clientele. This was followed quite naturally by the envy at least of his professional brethren. Feeling became so bitter, that even the possibility of serious personal consequences for him because of false accusations was not out of the question. Whenever novelties are introduced into medical science or medical practice, their authors are likely to meet with this opposition on the part of colleagues, and history is full of examples of it. Galvani was laughed at and called the frogs' dancing-master; Auenbrugger was made fun of for drumming on people; Harvey is said to have lost half of his consulting practice;—all because they were advancing ideas that their contemporaries were not ready to accept. We are rather likely to think that this intolerant attitude of mind belongs to the older times, but it is rather easy to trace it in our own.

In Constantine's day men had ready to hand a very serious weapon that might be used against innovators. By craftily circulated rumors the populace was brought to accuse him of magical practices, that is, of producing his cures by association with the devil. We are rather prone to think little of a generation that could take such nonsense seriously, but it would not be hard to find analogous false notions prevalent at the present time, which sometimes make life difficult, if not dangerous, for well-meaning individuals.[10] Life seems to have been made very uncomfortable for Constantine in Carthage. Just the extent to which persecution went, however, we do not know. About this time Constantine's work attracted the attention of Duke Robert of Salerno. He invited him to become his physician. After he had filled the position for a time a personal friendship developed, and, as has often happened to the physicians of kings, he became a royal counsellor and private secretary. When the post of professor of medicine at Salerno fell vacant, it is not surprising, then, that Constantine should have been made professor, and from here his teaching soon attracted the attention of all the men of his time.

Constantine seems to have greatly enhanced the reputation of the medical school, and added to the medical prestige of Salerno. After teaching for some ten years there, however, he gave up his professorship – the highest position in the medical world of the time – apparently with certain plans in mind.He wanted leisure for writing the many things in medicine that he had learned in his travels in the East, so as to pass his precious treasure of knowledge on to succeeding generations; and then, too, he seems to have longed for that peace that would enable him not only to do his writing undisturbed, but to live his life quietly far away from the strife of men and the strenuous existence of a court and of a great school.

There was probably another and more intimate personal reason for his retirement. Abbot Desiderius of the Benedictine Abbey of Monte Cassino, not far away, had become a close and valued friend. Before having been made abbot, Desiderius and Constantine probably were fellow professors at Salerno, for we know that Desiderius himself and many of his fellow Benedictines taught in the undergraduate department there. Desiderius enjoyed the reputation of being one of the most learned men of the time when his election to the abbacy at Monte Cassino took him away from Salerno. His departure was a blow to Constantine, who had learned by years of friendship that to be near his intimate friend, the pious scholarly Benedictine, was a solace in life and a never failing incentive to his own intellectual work. Desiderius seems, indeed, to have been a large factor in influencing the great physician to write his books rather than devote himself to oral teaching, since the circulation of his writing would confer so much more of benefit on a greater number of people. Perhaps another element in the situation was that Desiderius was desirous of having the learned physician, the travelled scholar, at Monte Cassino, for the sake of his influence on the scholarship of the abbey, and for the incentive that he would be to the younger monks to apply themselves to the varied field of knowledge which the Benedictines had chosen for themselves at this time.

Whatever hopes of mutual solace and helpfulness and of the joys of intimate close friendship may have been in the minds of these two most learned men of their time, they were destined to be grievously disappointed. Only a few years after Constantine's entrance into the monastery at Monte Cassino Desiderius was elected Pope. The humble Benedictine did not want to take the exalted position, but it was plainly shown to him that it was his duty, and that he must not shirk it. Accordingly, under the name of Pope Victor III, he became one of the great Popes of the eleventh century. One might think that he could have summoned Constantine to Rome, but perhaps he knew that his friend would prefer the quietude of the cloister, and then, too, probably he wanted to allow him the opportunity to accomplish that writing for which Constantine and himself had planned when the great physician entered the monastery.

All that we know for sure is that some twenty years of Constantine's life were spent as a monk in Monte Cassino, where he devoted his time mainly to the writing of his books. One bond of union there was. Each of the works, as soon as completed, was sent off to the Pope as long as he lived. On the other hand, though busy with his Papal duties, Pope Victor constantly stimulated Constantine, even from distant Rome, to go on with his work. There were messages of brotherly interest and solicitude just as in the old days. The great African physician's best known work, the so-called "Liber Pantegni," which is really a translation of the "Khitaab el Maleki" of Ali Ben el-Abbas, is dedicated to Desiderius. Constantine wrote a number of other books, most of them original, but it is difficult now to decide just which of those that pass under his name are genuine. Many were subsequently attributed to him that are surely not his.

These translators of the Middle Ages proved to be not only the channels through which information came to their generations, but they were also incentives to study and investigation. It is when men can get a certain amount of information rather easily that they are tempted to seek further in order to solve the problems that present themselves. There are three great translators whose work meant much for the Middle Ages at this time. They were, besides Constantine in the eleventh century, Gerard of Cremona, in the twelfth, and the Jewish Faradj Ben Salim, at Naples, in the thirteenth. Gerard did in Spain for the greater Arabian writers what Constantine had accomplished for those of lesser import. Under the patronage of the Emperor Frederick Barbarossa, he published translations of Rhazes, Isaac Judæus, Serapion, Abulcasis, and Avicenna. His work was done in Toledo, the city in which, during the twelfth and thirteenth centuries, so many translators were at work making books for the Western world.

Constantine did much more than merely bring out his translations of Arabian works. He gave a zest to the study of the old masters, issued editions of certain, at least, of the works of Hippocrates ("Aphorisms") and Galen ("Microtechnics"), and, in general, called attention to the precious treasure of medical lore that must be used to advantage if men were to teach the rising generation out of the accumulated knowledge of the past. Pagel, in Puschmann's "Handbook," does not hesitate to say that "a farther merit of Constantine must be recognized, inasmuch as that not long after his career the second epoch of the school of Salerno begins, marked not only by a wealth of writers and writings on medicine, but, above all, because from this time on the study of Greek medicine received renewed encouragement through the Latin versions of the Arabian literature. We may think as we will of the worth of these works, but this much is sure, that in many ways they brought about a broadening and an improvement of Greek knowledge, especially from the pharmacopeia standpoint."

Probably the best evidence that we have for Constantine's influence on his generation is to be found in what was accomplished by men who acknowledged with pride that he was their master, and who thought it a mark of distinction to be reckoned as his disciples.

Among these especially noteworthy is Johannes Afflacius, or Saracenus (whose surname of the Saracen probably means that he, too, came from Africa, as his master did). He was the author of two treatises on "Fevers and Urines," and the so-called "Cures of Afflacius." Some of these cures he directly attributed to Constantine. Then there is a Bartholomew who wrote a "Practica," or "Manual of the Practice of Medicine," with the sub-title, "Introductions to and Experiments in the Medical Practice of Hippocrates, Constantine, and the Greek Physicians." Bartholomew represents himself as a disciple of Constantine. This "Practica" of Bartholomew was one of the most commonly used books of the twelfth and thirteenth centuries throughout Europe. There are manuscript commentaries and translations, and abstracts from it not only in the Latin tongues, but especially in the Teutonic languages. Pagel refers to manuscripts in High and Low Dutch, and even in Danish. The Middle High Dutch manuscripts of this

"Practica" of Bartholomew come mainly from the thirteenth century, and have not only a special interest because of their value in the history of philology, but because they are the main sources of all the later books on drugs which appeared in very large numbers in German. They have a very great historico-literary interest, especially for pharmacology.

To Afflacius we owe a description of a method of reducing fever that is not only ingenious, but, in the light of our recently introduced bathing methods for fever, is a little startling. In his book on "Fevers and Urines," Afflacius suggests that when the patient's fever makes him very restless, and especially if it is warm weather, a sort of shower bath should be given to him. He thought that rain water was the best for this purpose, and he describes its best application as in rainy fashion, *modo pluviali.* The water should be allowed to flow down over the patient from a vessel with a number of minute perforations in the bottom. A number of the practical hints for treatment given by Afflacius have been attributed to Constantine.

Constantine's reputation has, in the opinion of some writers, been hurt by two features of his published works, as they have come to us, that we find it difficult to understand. One of these is that his translations from the Arabic were made mainly not of the books of the great leaders of Arabian medicine, but from certain of the less important writers. The other is that it does not seem always to have been made clear in the manuscripts that have come down to us, whether these writings were translations or original writings. Some have even gone so far as to suggest that Constantine himself would have been quite willing to receive the credit for these writings.

As to the first of these objections, it may be said that very probably Constantine, in his travels, had come to realize that the books of the great Arabian physicians, Rhazes, Abulcasis, Avicenna, and others, already received so much attention that the best outlook for medicine was to call particular notice to the writings of such lesser lights as Ali Abbas, Isaac Judæus, Abu Dschafer, and others of even less note. Certainly we cannot but feel that his judgment in the matter must have been directed by reasons that we may not be able to understand at present, but that must have existed, for all that we know of the man proves his character as a practical, far-sighted scholar. Besides, it seems not unlikely that but for his interest in them we would not at the present time possess the translations of these minor Arabian writers, and that would be an unfortunate gap in medical history.

The other misunderstanding with regard to Constantine refers to the fact that it is now almost impossible to decide which are his own and which are the writings of others. It has been said that he even tried to palm off some of the writings of others as his own. This seems extremely unlikely, however, knowing all that we do about his life;

and the suspicion is founded entirely on manuscripts as we have them at the present time, about a thousand years after he lived. What mutilations these manuscripts underwent in the course of various copyings is hard now to estimate. Monastic copyists might very well have left out Arabian names, because they were mainly interested in the fact that they were providing for their readers works that had received the approval of Constantine, and the translation of which at least had been made under his direction. It is quite clear that he did not do all the translating himself, and that he probably must have organized a school of medical translators at Monte Cassino. Then just how the various works would be looked at is very dubious. Undoubtedly many of the translations were done after his death, or certainly finished after his time, and at last attributed to him, because he was the moving spirit and had probably selected the books that should be translated, and made suggestions with regard to them. For all of his monks he was, as masters have ever been for disciples, much more important, and rightly so, than those writers to whom he referred them.

The whole question of plagiarism in these medieval times, as I have pointed out elsewhere, is entirely different from that of the present time. Now a writer may consciously or unconsciously claim another writing as his own. We have come to a time when men think much of their individual reputations. It was no uncommon thing, however, in the Middle Ages, and even later in the Renaissance, for a writer to attribute what he had written to some distinguished literary man of the preceding time, and sign that writer's name to his own work. The idea of the later author was to secure an audience for his thoughts. He seemed to be quite indifferent whether people ever knew just who the writer was, but he wanted to influence humanity by his writings. He thought much more of this than of any possible reputation that might come to him. Of course, there was no question of money. There never has been any question of money-making whenever the things written have been really worth while. Literature that has deeply influenced mankind has never paid. Publications that have paid are insignificant works that have touched superficially a whole lot of people. To think of Constantine as a plagiarist in our modern sense of the word, as trying to take the credit for someone else's writings, is to misunderstand entirely the times in which he lived, and to ignore the real problem of plagiarism at that time.

With the accumulation of information with regard to the history of medicine in his time, Constantine's reputation has been constantly enhanced. It is not so long since he was considered scarcely more than a monkish chronicler, who happened to have taken medicine rather than history for his field of work. Gradually we have come to appreciate all that he did for the medicine of his time. Undoubtedly his extensive travels, his wide knowledge, and then his years of effort to make Oriental medicine available for the Western civilization that was springing up again among the peoples who had come to replace the Romans, set him among the great intellectual forces of the Middle Ages. Salerno owed much to him, and it must not be forgotten that Salerno was the first university of modern times, and, above all, the first medical school that raised the dignity of the medical profession, established standards of medical education, educated the public mind and the rulers of the time to the realization of the necessity for the regulation of the practice of medicine, and in many ways anticipated our modern professional life. That the better part of his life work should have been done as a Benedictine only serves to emphasize the place that the religious had in the preservation and the development of culture and of education during the Middle Ages.

VIII

MEDIEVAL WOMEN PHYSICIANS

Very probably the most interesting chapter for us of the modern time in the history of the medical school at Salerno is to be found in the opportunities provided for the medical education of women and the surrender to them of a whole department in the medical school, that of Women's Diseases. While it is probable that Salerno did not owe its origin to the Benedictines, and it is even possible that there was some medical teaching there for all the centuries of the Middle Ages from the Greek times, for it must not be forgotten that this part of Italy was settled by Greeks, and was often called Magna Græcia, there is no doubt at all that the Benedictines exercised great influence in the counsels of the school, and that many of the teachers were Benedictines, as were also the Archbishops, who were its best patrons, and the great Pope Victor III, who did much for it. For several centuries the Benedictines represented the most potent influence at Salerno.

For most people who are not intimately familiar with monastic life, and, above all, with the story of the Benedictines, their prestige at Salerno might seem to be enough of itself to preclude all possibility of the education of women in medicine at Salerno. For those who know the Benedictines well, however,such a departure as the accordance of opportunities for women to study medicine would seem eminently in keeping with the practical wisdom of their rules and the development of their work. From the beginning the Benedictines recognized that a monastic career should be open to women as well as to men, and Benedict's sister, Scholastica, established convents for them, as her brother did the Benedictine monasteries, thus providing a vocation for women who did not feel called upon to marry. That the members of the order should recognize the advisability of affording women the opportunity to study medicine, and of handing over to them the department of women's diseases in a medical school in which they had a considerable amount of authority, seems, then, indeed, only what might have been expected of them.

We are prone in the modern time to think that our generation is the first to offer to women any facilities or opportunities for education in medicine. We are prone, however, just in the same way, to consider that a number of things that we are doing are now being done for the first time. As a matter of fact, it is extremely difficult to find any important movement or occupation that is not merely a repetition of a previous interest of mankind. The whole question of feminine education we are apt to think of as modern, forgetting that Plato insisted in his "Republic," as absolutely as any modern feminist, that women should have the same opportunities for education as men, and that at Rome, at the end of the Republic and the beginning of the Empire, the women occupied very much the same position in social life as our own at the present time. Their husbands supplied the funds, and they patronized the artists, gave receptions to the poets, lionized the musicians, and, in general, "went after culture" in a way that is a startling reminder of what we are familiar with in our own time. Just as soon as Christianity began to influence education, women were given abundant opportunities for higher education in all forms. In Ireland, the first nation completely converted to Christianity,—where, therefore, the national policy in education could be shaped by the Church without hindrance,—St. Brigid's school at Kildare was scarcely less famous than St.

Patrick's at Armagh. It had several thousand students, and, to a certain extent at least, co-education existed. In Charlemagne's time, with the revival of education on the Continent, the women of the Imperial Court attended the Palace School, as well as the men. In the thirteenth century we find women professors in every branch at Italian universities. Some of them were at least assistants in anatomy. The Renaissance women were, of course, profoundly educated. In a word, we have many phases of feminine education, though with intervals of absolutely negative interest, down the centuries.

There had evidently been quite a considerable amount of opportunity, if not of actual encouragement, for women in medicine, both among the Greeks and the Romans, in the early centuries of the Christian era. Galen, for instance, quotes certain prescriptions from women physicians. One Cleopatra is said to have written a book on cosmetics. This name came afterwards to be confounded with that of Queen Cleopatra, giving new prestige to the book, but neither Galen nor Aëtius, the early Christian physician, both of whom quote from her work, speak of her as anything except a medical writer. Some monuments to women physicians from these old times have escaped the tooth of time. There was the tomb of one Basila, and also of a Thecla, both of whom are said to have been physicians. Two other names of Greek women physicians we have, Origenia and Aspasia, the former mentioned by Galen, the latter by Aëtius in his "Tetrabiblion." Daremberg, the medical historian, announced in 1851 that he had found a Greek manuscript with the title, "On Women's Diseases," written by one Metrodora, a woman physician. He promised to publish it. It was unpublished at the time of his death, but could not be found among his papers. There is a manuscript on medical subjects, bearing this name, mentioned in the catalogue of the Greek Codices of the Laurentian Library at Florence, but this is said to give no indication of the time when its author lived. We have evidence enough, however, to show that Greek women physicians were not very rare.

The Romans imitated the Greeks so faithfully—one might almost say copied them so closely—that it is not surprising to find a number of Roman women physicians. The first mention of them comes from Scribonius Largus, in the first century after Christ. Octavius Horatianus, whom most of us know better as Priscian, dedicated one of his books on medicine to a woman physician named Victoria. The dedication leaves no doubt that she was a woman in active practice, at least in women's diseases, and it is a book on this subject that Priscian dedicates to her. He mentions another woman physician, Leoparda. The word *medica* for a woman physician was very commonly used at Rome. Martial, whose epigrams have been a source of so much information in medical history, especially on subjects with regard to which information was scanty, mentions a *medica* in an epigram. Apuleius also uses the word. There are a number of inscriptions in which women physicians are mentioned. Among the Christians we find women physicians, and Theodosia, the mother of St. Procopius, the martyr, is said to have been very successful in the practice of both medicine and surgery. She is numbered among the martyrs, and occurs in the Roman Martyrology on the 29th of May. Father Bzowski, the Polish Jesuit, who compiled "Nomenclatura Sanctorum Professione Medicorum" (Rome, 1621; the book is usually catalogued under the Latin form of his name, Bzovius), has among his list of saints who were physicians by profession a woman, St. Nicerata, who lived at Constantinople in the reign of the Emperor Arcadius, and who is said to have cured St. John Chrysostom of a serious disease.

The organization of the department of women's diseases at Salerno, under the care of women professors, and the granting of licenses to women to practise medicine, is not so surprising in the light of this tradition among Greeks and Romans, taken up with some enthusiasm by the Christians. We are not sure just when this development took place. The first definite evidence with regard to it comes in the life of Trotula, who seems to have been the head of the department. Some of her books are well known, and often quoted from, and she contributed to a symposium on the treatment of disease, in which there are contributions, also, from men professors of Salerno at the time. She seems to have flourished about the middle of the eleventh century. Ordericus Vitalis, a monk of Utica, who wrote an ecclesiastical history, tells of one Rudolph Malcorona, who, in 1059, came to Utica and remained there for a long time with Father Robert, his nephew. "This Rudolph had been a student all his life, devoting himself with great zeal to letters, and had become famous for his visits to the schools of France and Italy, in order to gather there the secrets of learning. As a consequence he was well informed not only in grammar and dialectics, but also in astronomy and in music. He also possessed such an extensive knowledge of the natural sciences that in the town of Salerno, where, since ancient times, the best schools of medicine had existed, there was no one to equal him with the exception of a very wise matron."

This wise matron has been identified with Trotula, many of the details of whose life have been brought to light by De Renzi, in his "Story of the School of Salerno."[11] According to very old tradition, Trotula belonged to the family of Ruggiero. This was a noble family of Salerno, many of the members of which were distinguished in their native town at least, but the name is not unusual in Italy,as readers of Dante and Boccaccio are likely to know. It was, indeed, as common as our own Rogers, of which it is the Italian equivalent.

De Renzi has made out a rather good case for the tradition that Trotula was the wife of John Platearius I—so called because there were probably three professors of that name. Trotula was, according to this, the mother of the second

Platearius, and the grandmother of the third, all of them distinguished members of the faculty at Salerno.

Her reputation extended far beyond her native town, and even Italy itself, and, in later centuries, her name was used to dignify any form of treatment for women's diseases that was being exploited. Rutebeuf, one of the *trouvères,* thirteenth-century French poets, has a description of the scene in which one of the old herbalist doctors who used to go round and collect a crowd by means of songs and music, and then talk medicine to them—just as is done even yet in many of the smaller towns of this country—is represented as saying to the crowd when he wants to make them realize that he is no ordinary quacksalver, that he is one of the disciples of the great Madame Trot of Salerno. The old-fashioned speech runs somewhat as follows: "Charming people: I am not one of these poor preachers, nor the poor herbalists, who carry little boxes and sachets, and who spread out before them a carpet. I am the disciple of a great lady, who bears the name of Madame Trot of Salerno. And I would have you know that she is the wisest woman in all the four quarters of the world."

Two books are attributed to Trotula; one bears the title, "De Passionibus Mulierum," and the other has been called "Trotula Minor," or "Summula Secundum Trotulam," and is a compendium of what she wrote. This is probably due to some disciple, but seems to have existed almost in her own time. Her most important work bears two sub-titles, "Trotula's Unique Book for the Curing of Diseases of Women, Before, During, and After Labor," and the other sub-title, "Trotula's Wonderful Book of Experience (*experimentalis*) in the Diseases of Women, Before, During, and After Labor, with Other Details Likewise Relating to Labor."

The book begins with a prologue on the nature of man and of woman, and an explanation of how the author, taking pity on the sufferings of women, came to devote herself to the study of their diseases. There are many interesting details in the book, all the more interesting because in many ways they anticipate modern solutions of difficult problems in women's diseases, and the care of the mother and child before, during, and after labor. For instance, there are a series of rules on the choice of the nurse, and on the diet and the régime which she should follow if the child is to be properly nourished without disturbance.

Probably the most striking passage in her book is that with regard to a torn perineum and its repair. This passage may be found in De Renzi or in Gurlt. It runs as follows: "Certain patients, from the severity of the labor, run into a rupture of the genitalia. In some even the vulva and anus become one foramen, having the same course. As a consequence, prolapse of the uterus occurs, and it becomes indurated. In order to relieve this condition, we apply to the uterus warm wine in which butter has been boiled, and these fomentations are continued until the uterus becomes soft, and then it is gently replaced. After this the tear between the anus and vulva we sew in three or four places with silk thread. The woman should then be placed in bed, with the feet elevated, and must retain that position, even for eating and drinking, and all the necessities of life, for eight or nine days. During this time, also, there must be no bathing, and care must be taken to avoid everything that might cause coughing, and all indigestible materials."

There is a passage, also, almost more interesting with regard to prophylaxis of rupture of the perineum. She says, "In order to avoid the aforesaid danger, careful provision should be made, and precautions should be taken during labor somewhat as follows: A cloth should be folded in somewhat oblong shape, and placed on the anus, so that, during every effort for the expulsion of the child, that should be pressed firmly, in order that there may not be any solution of the continuity of tissue."

Her book contains, also, some directions for various cosmetics. How many of these are original, however, is difficult to say. Trotula's name had become a word to conjure with, and many a quack in the after time tried to make capital for his remedies in this line by attributing them to Trotula. As a consequence, many of these remedies gradually found their way into the manuscript copies of her book, and subsequent copyists incorporated them into the text, until it became practically impossible to determine which were original. There are manuscripts of Trotula's work in Florence, Vienna, and Breslau. Some of these contain chapters not in the others, undoubtedly added by subsequent hands. In one of these, that at Florence, from which the edition of Strasburg was printed in 1544, and of Venice, 1547, one of the Aldine issues, there is a mention in the last chapter of spectacles. We have no record of these until the end of the thirteenth century, when this passage was probably added. It was also printed at Basle, 1566, and at Leipzig as late as 1778, which would serve to show how much attention it has attracted even in comparatively recent times.

After Trotula we have a number of women physicians of Salerno whose names have come down to us. The best known of these bear the names Constanza, Calendula, Abella, Mercuriade, Rebecca Guarna, who belonged to the old Salernitan family of that name, a member of which, in the twelfth century, was Romuald, priest, physician, and historian, Louise Trencapilli, and others. The titles of some of their books, as those of Mercuriade, who occupied herself with surgery as well as medicine, and who is said to have written on "Crises," on "Pestilent Fever," on "The Cure of Wounds," and of Abella, who acquired a great reputation with her work on "Black Bile," and on the "Nature of Seminal Fluid," have come down to us. Rebecca Guarna wrote on "Fevers," on the "Urine," and on the "Embryo." The school of Salernitan women came to have a definite place in medical literature.

While, as teachers, they had charge of the department of women's diseases, their writings would seem to indicate that they studied all branches of medicine. Besides, there are a number of licenses preserved in the archives of Naples in which women are accorded the privilege of practising medicine. Apparently these licenses were without limitation. In many of these mention is made of the fact that it seems especially fitting that women should be allowed to practise in women's diseases, since they are by constitution likely to know more and to have more sympathy with feminine ills. The formula employed as the preamble of this license ran as follows: "Since, then, the law permits women to exercise the profession of physicians, and since, besides, due regard being had to purity of morals, women are better suited for the treatment of women's diseases, after having received the oath of fidelity, we permit, etc."

Salerno continued to enjoy a reputation for training women physicians thoroughly, until well on in the fifteenth century, for we have the record of Constance Calenda, the daughter of Salvator Calenda, who had been dean of the faculty of medicine at Salerno about 1415, and afterwards dean of the faculty at Naples. His daughter, under the diligent instruction of her father, seems to have obtained special honors for her medical examination. Not long after this, Salerno itself lost all the prestige that it had. The Kings of Naples endeavored to create a great university in their city in the thirteenth century. They did not succeed to the extent that they hoped, but the neighboring rival institution hurt Salerno very much, and its downfall may be traced from this time. Gradually its reputation waned, and we have practically no medical writer of distinction there at the end of the fourteenth century, though the old custom of opportunities for women students of medicine was maintained.

This custom seems also to have been transferred to Naples, and licenses to practise were issued to woman graduates of Naples. This never achieved anything like the reputation in this department that had been attained at Salerno. Salerno influenced Bologna and the north Italian universities profoundly in all branches of medicine and medical education, particularly in surgery, as can be seen in the chapter on "Great Surgeons of the Medieval Universities," and the practice of allowing such women as wished to study medicine to enter the university medical schools is exemplified in the case of Mondino's assistant in anatomy, Alessandra Giliani, though there are also others whose names have come down to us.

The University of Salerno had developed round a medical school. It was the first of the universities, and, in connection with its medical school, feminine education obtained a strong foothold. It is not surprising, then, that with the further development of universities in Italy, feminine education came to be the rule. This rule has maintained itself all down the centuries in Italy, so that there has not been a single century since the twelfth in which there have not been one or more distinguished women teachers at the Italian universities. University life gradually spread westward, and Paris came into existence as an organized institution of learning after Bologna, and, doubtless, with some of the traditions of Salerno in the minds of its founders. Feminine education, however, did not spread to the West. This is a little bit difficult to understand, considering the reverence that the Teutonic peoples have always had for their women folk and the privileges accorded them. A single unfortunate incident, that of Abélard and Héloïse, seems to have been sufficient to discourage efforts in the direction of opportunities for feminine education in connection with the Western universities. Perhaps, in the less sophisticated countries of the North and West of Europe, women did not so ardently desire educational opportunities as in Italy, for whenever they have really wanted them, as, indeed, anything else, they have always obtained them.

In spite of the absence of formal opportunities for feminine education in medicine at the Western universities, a certain amount of scientific knowledge of diseases, as well as valuable practical training in the care of the ailing, was not wanting for women outside of Italy. The medical knowledge of the women of northern France and Germany and England, however, though it did not receive the stamp of a formal degree from the university and the distinction of a license to practise, was none the less thorough and extensive. It came in connection with certain offices in their own communities, held by members of religious orders. Genuine information with regard to what the religious were doing during the Middle Ages was so much obscured by the tradition of laziness and immorality, created at the time of the so-called reformation in order to justify the confiscation of their property by those whose one object was to enrich themselves, that we have only come to know the reality of their life and accomplishments in comparatively recent years. We now know that, besides being the home of most of the book knowledge of the earlier Middle Ages, the monasteries were the constant patrons of such practical subjects as architecture, agriculture in all its phases, especially irrigation, draining, and the improvement of land and crops; of art, and even what we now know as physical science. Above all, they preserved for us the old medical books and carried on medical traditions of practice. The greatest surprise has been to find that this was true not only for the monks, but also for the nuns.

One of the most important books on medicine that has come to us from the twelfth century is that of a Benedictine abbess, since known as St. Hildegarde, whose life was spent in the Rhineland. Her works serve to show very well that in the convents of the tenth, eleventh, and twelfth centuries there was much more of interest in things intellectual than we have had any idea of until recent years, and that, indeed, one of the important occupations of convent life was the serious study of books of all kinds, some of them even scientific, as well as the writing of works in all departments. The century before St. Hildegarde there is the record of Hroswitha, who wrote a series of dramas in imitation of Terence, that were meant to replace, for the monks and nuns of that period, the reading of that rather too human author. Hroswitha, like Hildegarde, was a German, and we have the record, also, of another religious writer, abbess of the Odilian Cloister, at Hohenberg, who wrote a book called "Hortus Deliciarum, the Garden of Delights," a book of information on many subjects not unlike our popular encyclopedias of the modern time, the title of which shows that the place of information in life was considered to be the giving of pleasure. While this work deals mainly with Biblical and theological and mystical questions, there are many purely scientific passages and many subjects of strictly medical interest treated.

The life of the Abbess Hildegarde is worthy of consideration, because it illustrates the period and makes it very clear that, in spite of the grievous misunderstanding of their life and work, so common in the modern time, these old-time religious had most of the interests of the modern time, and pursued them with even more than modern zeal and success, very often. Her career illustrates very well what the foundation of the Benedictines had done for women. When St. Benedict founded his order for men, his sister, Scholastica, wanted to do a similar work for women. We know that the Benedictine monks saved the old classics for us, kept burning the light of the intellectual life, and gave a refuge to men who wanted to devote themselves in leisure and peace to the things of the spirit, whether of this world or the other. We have known much less of the Benedictine nuns until now the study of their books shows that they provided exactly the same opportunities for women and furnished a vocation, a home, an occupation of mind, and a satisfaction of spirit for the women who, in every generation, do not feel themselves called to be wives and mothers, but who want to live their lives for others rather than for themselves and their kin, seeking such development of mind and of spirit as may come with the leisure and peace of celibacy.

Hildegarde was born of noble parents at Böckelheim, in the county of Sponheim, about the end of the eleventh century (probably 1098). In her eighth year she went for her education to the Benedictine cloister of Disibodenberg. When her education was finished, she entered the cloister, of which, at the age of about fifty, she became abbess. Her writings, reputation for sanctity, and her wise saintly rule attracted so many new members to the community that the convent became overcrowded. Accordingly, with eighteen of her nuns, Hildegarde withdrew to a new convent at Rupertsberg, which English and American travellers will remember because it is not far from Bingen on the Rhine. Here she came to be a centre of attraction for most of the world of her time. She was in active correspondence with nearly every important man of her generation. She was an intimate friend of Bernard of Clairvaux, who was himself, perhaps, the most influential man in Europe in this century. She was in correspondence with four Popes, and with the Emperors Conrad and Frederick I, and with many distinguished archbishops, abbots, and abbesses, and teachers and teaching bodies of various kinds. These correspondences were usually begun by her correspondents, who consulted her because her advice in difficult problems was considered so valuable.

In spite of all this time-taking correspondence, she found leisure to write a series of books, most of them on mystical subjects, but two of them on medical subjects. The first is called "Liber Simplicis Medicinæ," and the second "Liber Compositæ Medicinæ." These books were written in order to provide information mainly for the nuns who had charge of the infirmaries of the monasteries of the Benedictines. Almost constantly someone in the large communities, which always contained aged religious, was ailing, and then, besides, there were other calls on the time and the skill of the sister infirmarians. There were no hotels at that time, and no hospitals, except in the large cities. There were always guest houses in connection with monasteries and convents, in which travellers were permitted to pass the night, and given what they needed to eat. There are many people who have had experiences of monastic hospitality even in our own time. Sometimes travellers fell ill. Not infrequently the reason for travelling was to find health in some distant and fabulously health-giving resort, or at the hands of some wonder-working physician. Such high hopes are nearly always set at a distance. This of itself must have given not a little additional need for knowledge of medicine to the infirmarians of convents and monasteries. There were around many of the monasteries, moreover, large estates; often they had been cleared and made valuable by the work of preceding generations of monks, and on these estates peasants came to live. Workingmen and workingwomen from neighboring districts came to help at harvest time, and, after a chance meeting, were married and settled down on a little plot of ground provided for them near the monastery. As these communities grew up, they looked to the monasteries and convents for aid of all kinds, and turned to them particularly in times of illness. The need for definite instruction in medicine on the part of a great many of the monks and nuns can be readily understood, and it was this need that Hildegarde tried to meet in her books. The first of her books that we have mentioned, the "Liber Simplicis Medicinæ," attracted attention rather early in the Renaissance, and was deemed worthy of print. It was edited at the beginning of the sixteenth century by Dr. Schott at Strasburg, under the title, "Physica S. Hildegardis." Another manuscript of this part was found in the library of Wolfenbuttel, in 1858, by Dr. Jessen. This gave him an interest in Hildegarde's contributions to medicine, and, in 1859, he noted in the library at Copenhagen a manuscript with the title "Hildegardi Curæ et Causæ." On examination, he was sure that it was the "Liber Compositæ Medicinæ" of the saint. The first work consists of nine books, treating of plants, elements, trees, stones, fishes, birds, quadrupeds, reptiles, and metals, and is printed in Migne's "Patrologia," under the title "Subtilitatum Diversarum Naturarum Libri Novem." The second, in five books, treats of the general diseases of created things, of the human body and its ailments, of the causes, symptoms, and treatment of diseases.

It would be very easy to think that these are small volumes and that they contain very little. We are so apt to think of old-fashioned so-called books as scarcely more than chapters, that it may be interesting to give some idea of the contents and extent of the first of these works. The first book on Plants has 230 chapters, the second on the Elements has 13 chapters, the third on Trees has 36 chapters, the fourth on various kinds of Minerals, including precious stones, has 226 chapters, the fifth on Fishes has 36 chapters, the sixth on Birds has 68 chapters, the seventh on Quadrupeds has 43 chapters, the eighth on Reptiles has 18 chapters, the ninth on Metals has 8 chapters. Each chapter begins with a description of the species in question, and then defines its value for man and its therapeutic significance. Modern scientists have not hesitated to declare that the descriptions abound in observations worthy of a scientific inquiring spirit. We are, of course, not absolutely sure that all the contents of the books come from Hildegarde. Subsequent students often made notes in these manuscript books, and then other copyists copied these into the texts. Unfortunately we have not a number of codices to collate and correct such errors. Most of what Hildegarde wrote comes to us in a single copy, of none are there more than four copies, showing how near we came to missing all knowledge of her entirely.

Dr. Melanie Lipinska, in her "Histoire des Femmes Médecins," a thesis presented for the doctorate in medicine at the University of Paris in 1900, subsequently awarded a special prize by the French Academy, reviews Hildegarde's work critically from the medical standpoint. She says that the saint distinguishes a double mode of action of different substances, one chemical, the other physical, or what we would very probably call magnetic. She discusses all the ailments of the various organs, the brain, the eyes, the teeth, the heart, the spleen, the stomach, the liver. She has special chapters on redness and paleness of the face, on asthma, on cough, on fetid breath, on bilious indigestion, on gout. Besides, she has other chapters on nervous affections, on icterus, on fevers, on intestinal worms, on infections due to swamp exhalations, on dysentery, and a number of forms of pulmonary diseases. Nearly all of our methods of diagnosis are to be found, hinted at at least, in her book. She discusses the redness of the blood as a sign of health, the characteristics of various excrementitious material as signs of disease, the degrees of fever, and the changes in the pulse. Of course, it was changes in the humors of the body that constituted the main causes for disease in her opinion, but it is well to remind ourselves that our frequent discussion of auto-intoxication in recent years is a distinct return to this.

Some of Hildegarde's anticipations of modern ideas are, indeed, surprising enough. For instance, in talking about the stars and describing their course through the firmament, she makes use of a comparison that is rather startling. She says: "Just as the blood moves in the veins which causes them to vibrate and pulsate, so the stars move in the firmament and send out sparks as it were of light like the vibrations of the veins." This is, of course, not an anticipation of the discovery of the circulation of the blood, but it shows how close were men's ideas to some such thought five centuries before Harvey's discovery. For Hildegarde the brain was the regulator of all the vital qualities, the centre of life. She connects the nerves in their passage from the brain and the spinal cord through the body with manifestations of life. She has a series of chapters with regard to psychology normal and morbid. She talks about frenzy, insanity, despair, dread, obsession, anger, idiocy, and innocency. She says very strongly in one place that "when headache and migraine and vertigo attack a patient simultaneously they render a man foolish and upset his reason. This makes many people think that he is possessed of a demon, but that is not true." These are the exact words of the saint as quoted in Mlle. Lipinska's thesis.

It is no wonder that Mlle. Lipinska thinks St. Hildegarde the most important medical writer of her time. Reuss, the editor of the edition of Hildegarde published in Migne's "Patrology," says: "Among all the saintly religious who have practised medicine or written about it in the Middle Ages, the most important is without any doubt St. Hildegarde...." With regard to her book he says: "All those who wish to write the history of the medical and natural sciences must read this work in which this religious woman, evidently well grounded in all that was known at that time in the secrets of nature, discusses and examines carefully all the knowledge of the time." He adds, "It is certain that St. Hildegarde knew many things that were unknown to the physicians of her time."

When such books were read and widely copied, it shows that there was an interest in practical and scientific medicine among women in Germany much greater than is usually thought to have existed at this time. Such writers, though geniuses, and standing above their contemporaries, usually represent the spirit of their times and make it clear that definite knowledge of things medical was considered of value. The convents and monasteries of this time are often thought of by those who know least about them as little interested in anything except their own ease and certain superstitious practices. As a matter of fact, they cared for their estates, and especially for the peasantry on them, they provided lodging and food for travellers, they took care of the ailing of their neighborhood, and, besides, occupied themselves with many phases of the intellectual life. It was a well-known tradition that country people who lived in the neighborhood of convents and monasteries, and especially those who had monks and nuns for their landlords, were much happier and were much better taken care of than the tenantry of other estates. For this a cultivation of medical knowledge was necessary in certain, at least, of the members of the religious orders, and such books as Hildegarde's are the evidence that not only the knowledge existed, but that it was collected and written down, and widely disseminated.

Nicaise, in the introduction to his edition of Guy de Chauliac's "Grande Chirurgie," reviews briefly the history of women in medicine, and concludes:

> "Women continued to practise medicine in Italy for centuries, and the names of some who attained great renown have been preserved for us. Their works are still quoted from in the fifteenth century.
>
> "There was none of them in France who became distinguished, but women could practise medicine in certain towns at least on condition of passing an examination before regularly appointed masters. An edict of 1311, at the same time that it interdicts unauthorized

women from practising surgery, recognizes their right to practise the art if they have undergone an examination before the regularly appointed master surgeons of the corporation of Paris. An edict of King John, April, 1352, contains the same expressions as the previous edict. Du Bouley, in his 'History of the University of Paris,' gives another edict by the same King, also published in the year 1352, as a result of the complaints of the faculties at Paris, in which there is also question of women physicians. This responded to the petition: 'Having heard the petition of the Dean and the Masters of the Faculty of Medicine at the University of Paris, who declare that there are very many of both sexes, some of the women with legal title to practise and some of them merely old pretenders to a knowledge of medicine, who come to Paris in order to practise, be it enacted,' etc. (The edict then proceeds to repeat the terms of previous legislation in this matter.)

"Guy de Chauliac speaks also of women who practised surgery. They formed the fifth and last class of operators in his time. He complains that they are accustomed to too great an extent to give over patients suffering from all kinds of maladies to the will of Heaven, founding their practice on the maxim 'The Lord has given as he has pleased; the Lord will take away when he pleases; may the name of the Lord be blessed.'

"In the sixteenth century, according to Pasquier, the practice of medicine by women almost entirely disappeared. The number of women physicians becomes more and more

> rare in the following centuries just in proportion as we approach our own time. Pasquier says that we find a certain number of them anxious for knowledge and with a special penchant for the study of the natural sciences and even of medicine, but very few of them take up practice."

Just how the lack of interest in medical education for women gradually deepened, until there was almost a negative phase of it, only a few women in Italy devoting themselves to medicine, is hard to say. It is one of the mysteries of the vicissitudes of human affairs that ups and downs of interest in things practical as well as intellectual keep constantly occurring. The number of discoveries and inventions in medicine and surgery that we have neglected until they were forgotten, and then had to make again, is so well illustrated in chapters of this book, that I need only recall them here in general. It may seem a little harder to understand that so important a manifestation of interest in human affairs as the education and licensure of women physicians should not only cease, but pass entirely out of men's memory, yet such apparently was the case. It would not be hard to illustrate, as I have shown in "Cycles of Feminine Education and Influence" in "Education, How Old the New" (Fordham University Press, 1910), that corresponding ups and downs of interest may be traced in the history of feminine education of every kind. In that chapter I have discussed the possible reasons for these vicissitudes, which have no place here, but I may refer those who are interested in the subject to that treatment of it.

IX

MONDINO AND THE MEDICAL SCHOOL OF BOLOGNA

The most important contributions to medical science made by the Medical School of Salerno at the height of its development were in surgery. The text-books written by men trained in her halls or inspired by her teachers were to influence many succeeding generations of surgeons for centuries. Salerno's greatest legacy to Bologna was the group of distinguished surgical teachers whose text-books we have reviewed in the chapter, "Great Surgeons of the Medieval Universities." Bologna herself was to win a place in medical history, however, mainly in connection with anatomy, and it was in this department that she was to provide incentive especially for her sister universities of north Italy, though also for Western Europe generally. The first manual of dissection, that is, the first handy volume giving explicit directions for the dissection of human cadavers, was written at Bologna. This was scattered in thousands of copies in manuscript all over the medical world of the fourteenth and early fifteenth centuries. Even after the invention of printing, many editions of it were printed. Down to the sixteenth century it continued to be the most used text-book of anatomy, as well as manual of dissection, which students of every university had in hand when they made their dissection, or wished to prepare for making it, or desired to review it after the body had been taken away, for with lack of proper preservative preparation, bodies had to be removed in a comparatively short time. Probably no man more influenced the medical teaching of the fourteenth and fifteen centuries than Mundinus, or, as he was called in the Italian fashion, Mondino, who wrote this manual of dissection.

Mundinus quem omnis studentium universitas colit ut deum (Mundinus, whom all the world of students cultivated as a god), is the expression by which the German scholar who edited, about 1500, the Leipzig edition of Mundinus' well-known manual, the *Anathomia,* introduces it to his readers. The expression is well worth noting, because it shows what was still the reputation of Mundinus in the medical educational world nearly two centuries after his death.[12]

Until the time of Vesalius, whose influence was exerted about the middle of the sixteenth century, Mondino was looked up to by all teachers as the most important contributor to the science of anatomy in European medicine since the Greeks. He owed his reputation to two things: his book, of which we have already spoken, and then, the fact that he reintroduced dissection demonstrations as a regular practice in the medical schools. His book is really a manual of making anatomical preparations for demonstration purposes. These demonstrations had to be hurried, owing to the rapid decomposition of material consequent upon the lack of preservatives. The various chapters were prepared with the idea of supplying explicit directions and practical help during the anatomical demonstrations, so that these might be made as speedily as possible. The book does not comprise much that was new at that time, but it is a good compendium of previous knowledge, and contains some original observations. It was entirely owing to its form as a handy manual of anatomical knowledge and, besides, because it was an incentive to the practice of human dissection, that it attained and maintained its popularity.

Mondino followed Galen, of course, and so did every other teacher in medicine and its allied sciences, until Vesalius' time. Even Vesalius permitted himself to be influenced overmuch by Galen at points where we wonder that he did not make his observations for himself, since, apparently, they were so obvious. The more we know of Galen, however, the less surprised are we at his hold over the minds of men. Only those who are ignorant of Galen's immense knowledge, his practical common sense, and the frequent marvellous anticipations of what we think most modern, affect to despise him.His works have never been translated into any modern language except piecemeal, there is no complete translation, and one must be ready to delve into some large Latin, if not Greek, volumes to know what a marvel of medical knowledge he was, and how wise were the men who followed him closely, though, being human, there are times when necessarily he failed them.

For those who know even a little at first hand of Galen, it is only what might be expected, then, that Mondino, trying to break away from the anatomy of the pig, which had been before this the basis of all anatomical teaching in the medical schools (Copho's book, used at Salerno and Bologna before Mondino's was founded on dissections of the pig), should have clung somewhat too closely to this old Greek teacher and Greek master. The incentive furnished by Mondino's book helped to break the tradition of Galen's unquestioned authority. Besides this, the group of men around Mondino, his master, Taddeo Alderotti, with his disciples and assistants, form the initial chapter in the history of the medical school of Bologna, which gradually assumed the place of Salerno at this time. There is no better way of getting a definite idea of what was being done in medicine, and how it was being done, than by knowing some of the details of the life of this group of medical workers.

Mondino di Liucci, or Luzzi, is usually said to have been born about 1275. His first name is a diminutive for Raimondo. It used to be said of him that, like many of the great men of history, many cities claimed to be his birthplace. Five were particularly mentioned – Florence, Milan, Bologna, Forli, and Friuli. There is, however, another Mondino, a distinguished physician, who was born and lived at Friuli, and it is because of confusion with him that the claim for Friuli has been set up. Florence and Milan are considered out of the question. Mondino was probably born in or near Bologna. The fact that there should have been this multiple set of claims shows how much was thought of him. Indeed, his was the best known name in the medical schools of Europe for nearly two centuries and a half. He seems to have been a particularly brilliant student, for tradition records that he had obtained his degree of doctor of medicine when he was scarcely more than twenty. This seems quite out of the question for us at the present time, but we have taken to pushing back the time of graduation, and it is not sure whether this is, beyond peradventure, so beneficial as is usually thought.

That his early graduation did not hamper his intellectual development, the fact that, in 1306, when he was about thirty-one years of age, he was offered the professorial chair in anatomy, which he continued to occupy with such distinction for the next twenty years, would seem to prove. His public dissections of human bodies, probably the first thus regularly made, attracted widespread attention, and students came to him not only from all over Italy, but also from Europe generally. In this, after all, Mondino was only continuing the tradition of world teaching that Bologna had acquired under her great surgeons in the preceding century. (See "Great Surgeons of the Medieval Universities.")

Mondino came from a family that had already distinguished itself in medicine at Bologna. His uncle was a professor of physic at the university. His father, Albizzo di Luzzi, seems to have come from Florence not long after the middle of the thirteenth century, for the records show that, about 1270, he formed a partnership with one Bartolommeo Raineri for the establishment of a pharmacy at Bologna. Later this passed entirely under the control of the Mondino family, and came to be known as the Spezieria del Mondino. In it were sold, besides Eastern perfumes, spices, condiments, probably all sorts of toilet articles, and even rugs and silks and feminine ornaments. The stricter pharmacy of the earlier times developed into a sort of department store, something like our own. The Mondini, however, insisted always on the pharmacy feature as a specialty, and the fact was made patent to the general public by a sign with the picture of a doctor on it. This drug shop of the Mondini continued to be maintained as such, according to Dr. Pilcher, until the beginning of the nineteenth century.[13]

One of the fellow students of Mondino at the University of Bologna had been Mondeville. He came from distant France to take a course in surgery with Theodoric, whose high reputation in the olden time, vague with us half a century ago, is now amply justified by what we know of him from such ardent students and admirers as Pagel and Nicaise. Not long after Mondino's death, Guy de Chauliac came from France to reap similar opportunities to these, which had proved so fruitful for Mondeville. The more that we learn about this time the more do we find to make it clear how deeply interested the generation was in education in every form, artistic, philosophic, but, also, though this is often not realized, scientific.

The long distances, so much longer in that time than in ours, to which men were willing, and even anxious, to go, in order to obtain opportunities for research, and to get in touch with a special master, the associations with stimulating fellow pupils of other lands, the scientific correspondences, almost necessarily initiated by such circumstances, all indicate an enthusiasm for knowledge such as we have not been accustomed to attribute to this period. On the contrary, we have been rather inclined to think them neglectful of all education, and have, above all, listened acquiescently while men deprecated the lack of interest in things scientific displayed by these generations. Indeed, many writers have gone out of their way to find a reason for the supposed lack of interest in science at this time, and have proclaimed the Church's opposition to scientific education and study as the cause.

At this time Italy was the home of the graduate teaching for all Europe. The Italian Peninsula continued to be the foster-mother of the higher education in letters and art, but also, though this is less generally known, in science, for the next five centuries. Germany has come to be the place of pilgrimage for those who want higher opportunities in science than can be afforded in their own country only during the latter half of the nineteenth century. France occupied it during the first half of the nineteenth century. Except for short intervals, when political troubles disturbed Italy, as about the middle of the fourteenth century, when the removal of the Popes to Avignon brought their influence for education over to France and a short period at the beginning of the eighteenth century, when the Netherlands for a time came into educational prominence, Italy has always been the European Mecca for advanced students. Practically all our great discoverers in medicine, until the last century, were either Italians, or else had studied in Italy. Mondino, Bertruccio, Salicet, Lanfranc, Baverius, Berengarius, John De Vigo, who first wrote on gun-shot wounds; John of Arcoli, first to mention gold filling and other anticipations of modern dentistry; Varolius, Eustachius, Cæsalpinus, Columbus, Malpighi, Lancisi, Morgagni, Spallanzani, Galvani, Volta, were all Italians. Mondeville, Guy de Chauliac, Linacre, Vesalius, Harvey, Steno, and many others who might be named, all studied in Italy, and secured their best opportunities to do their great work there.

It would be amusing, if it were not amazing, to have serious writers of history in the light of this plain story of graduate teaching of science in Italy for over five centuries, write about the opposition of the Church to science during the Medieval and Renaissance periods. It is particularly surprising to have them talk of Church opposition to the medical sciences. The universities of the world all had their charters from the Popes at this time, and were all ruled by ecclesiastics, and most of the students and practically all of the professors down to the end of the sixteenth century belonged to the clerical order. The universities of Italy were all more directly under the control of ecclesiastical authority than anywhere else, and nearly all of them were dominated by papal influence. Bologna, while doing much of the best graduate work in science, especially in medicine, was, in the Papal States, absolutely under the rule of the Popes. The university was, practically, a department of the Papal government. The medical school at the University of Rome itself was for several centuries, at the end of the Middle Ages, the teaching-place where were assembled the pick of the great medical investigators, who, having reached distinction by their discoveries elsewhere, were summoned to Rome in order to add prestige to the Papal University. All of them became special friends of the Popes, dedicated their books to them, and evidently looked to them as beneficent patrons and hearty encouragers of original scientific research.

While this is so strikingly true of medical science as to make contrary declarations in the matter utterly ridiculous, and to suggest at once that there must be some motive for seeing things so different to the reality, the same story can be told of graduate science in other departments. It was to Italy that men came for special higher studies in mathematics and astronomy, in botany, in mineralogy, and in applied chemistry, so far as it related to the arts of painting, illuminating, stained-glass making, and the like. No student of science felt that he had quite exhausted the opportunities for study that were possible for him until he had been down in Italy for some time. To meet the great professors in Italy was looked on as sure to be a source of special incentive in any department of science. This is coming to be generally recognized just in proportion as our own interest in the arts and crafts, and in the history of science, leads us to go carefully into the details of these subjects at first hand. The editors of the "Cambridge Modern History," in their preface, declared ten years ago that we can no longer accept with confidence the declaration of any secondary writer on history. This is particularly true of the medieval period. We must go back to the writers of those times.

If it seems surprising that the University of Bologna should have come into such great prominence as an institute for higher education at this time, it would be well to recall some of the great work that is being done in this part of Italy in other departments at this time. Cimabue laid the foundation of modern art towards the end of the thirteenth century, and during Mondino's life Giotto, his pupil, raised an artistic structure that is the admiration of all generations of artists since. Dante's years are almost exactly contemporary with those of Giotto and of Mondino. If men were doing such wondrous work in literature and in art, why should not the same generation produce a man who will accomplish for the practical science of medicine what his friends and contemporaries had done in other great intellectual departments.

In recent years we have come to think much more of environment as an influence in human development and accomplishment than was the custom sometime ago. The broader general environment in Italy, with genius at work in other departments, was certainly enough to arouse in younger minds all their powers of original work. The narrower environment at Bologna itself was quite as stimulating, for a great clinical teacher, Taddeo Alderotti, had come, in 1260, from Florence to Bologna, to take up there the practice and teaching of medicine. It was under him that Mondino was to be trained for his life work.

To understand the place of Mondino, and of the medical school of Bologna, in his time, and the reputation that came to them as world teachers of medicine, we must know, first, this great teacher of Mondino and the atmosphere of progressive medicine that enveloped the university in the latter half of the thirteenth century. In the chapter on "Great Surgeons of the Medieval Universities" we call particular attention to the series of distinguished men, the first four of whom were educated at Salerno, and who came to Bologna to teach surgery. They were doing the best surgery in the world, much better than was done in many centuries after their time; indeed, probably better than at any period down to our own day. Besides, they seem to have been magnetic teachers who attracted and inspired pupils.We have the surgical contributions of a series of men, written at Bologna, that serve to show what fine work was accomplished. At this time, however, the field of medicine was not neglected, though we have but a single great historical name in it that has lived. This was Taddeo Alderotti, a man who lifted the medical profession as high in the estimation of his fellow citizens at Florence as the great painters and literary men of his time did their departments, and who then moved to Bologna, because of the opportunity to teach afforded him by the university.

It is sometimes a little difficult for casual students of the time to understand the marvellous reputation acquired by this medieval physician. It should not be, however, when we recall the enthusiastic reception and procession of welcome accorded to Cimabue's Madonna, and the almost universal acclaim of the greatness of Dante's work, even in his own time. In something of that same spirit Bologna came to appreciate Taddeo, as he is familiarly known, looked upon him as a benefactor of the community, and voted to relieve him of the burden of paying taxes. He came to be considered as a public institution, whose presence was a blessing to his fellow citizens, and whose goodness to them should be recognized in this public way. One is not surprised to hear Villani, the well-known contemporary historian, speak of him as the greatest physician in Christendom.

The feelings of the citizens of Bologna, it may well be confessed, were not entirely unselfish, or due solely to the desire to encourage a great scientific genius. Few men of his generation had done more for the city in a material way quite apart from whatever benefits he conferred upon the health of its citizens than Dr. Taddeo. It was he who organized medical teaching in the city on such a plane that it attracted students from all over the world. Bologna had had a great law school before this, founded by Irnerius, to which students had come from all over the world. With the advent of Taddeo from Florence, and his success as a medical practitioner, there began to flock to his lectures many students who spread his fame far and wide. The city council could scarcely do less than grant the same privileges to the medical students and teachers of Taddeo's school as they had previously accorded to the faculty of law and its students. The city council recognized quite as clearly as any board of aldermen in the modern time how much, even of material benefit, a great university was to the building up of a city, though their motives were probably much higher than that, and their enlightened policy had its reward in the rapid growth of Bologna until, very probably at the end of the thirteenth century, it had more students than any university of the modern time. The number was not less than fifteen thousand, and may have been twenty thousand.

To this great university success Taddeo and his medical school contributed not a little. The especially attractive feature of his teaching seems to have been its eminent practicalness. He himself had made an immense success of the practice of medicine, and accumulated a great fortune, so much so that Dante, in his "Paradiso," when he wishes to find a figure that would represent exactly the opposite to what St. Dominic, the founder of the Dominicans, did for the love of wisdom and humanity, he takes that of Taddeo, who had accomplished so much for personal reputation and wealth.

This might easily lead to the impression that Taddeo's teaching was unscientific, or merely empiric, or that he himself was a narrow-minded maker of money, intent only on his immediate influence, and hampered by exclusive devotion to practical medicine. Nothing could be farther from the truth than any such impression. Taddeo was not only the head of a great medical school, a great teacher whom his students almost worshipped, a physician to whom patients flocked because of his marvellous success, a fine citizen of a great city, whom his fellow citizens honored, but he was a broad-minded scholar, a philosopher, and even an author in branches apart from medicine.

In that older time it was the custom to combine the study of philosophy and medicine. For centuries after that period in Italy it was the custom for men to take both degrees, the doctorate in philosophy and in medicine at the same time. Indeed, most of those whose work has made them famous, down to and including Galvani, did so. Taddeo wrote commentaries on the works of Hippocrates and Galen, but he also translated the ethics of Aristotle, and did much to make the learning of the Arabs easily available for his students. His was a broad, liberal scholarship. Dr. Lewis Pilcher,in his article on "The Mondino Myth,"[14] does not hesitate to say that "to the spirit which, from his professorial chair, Taddeo infused into the teaching and study of medicine undoubtedly is due the high position which for many generations thereafter the school of Bologna continued to maintain as a centre of medical teaching."

Of course, erudition had its revenge, and carried Taddeo too far. The difficult thing in human nature is to stay in the mean and avoid exaggeration. His methods of illustrating medical truths from many literary and philosophical sources often caused the kernel of observation to be hidden beneath a blanket of speculation or, at least, to be concealed to a great extent. Even the Germans, who have insisted most on this unfortunate tendency of Taddeo, have been compelled to confess that there is much that is valuable in what he accomplished, and that even his modes of expression were not without a certain vivacity which attracted attention and doubtless added materially to his success as a teacher. Pagel, in Puschmann's "Handbuch," says: "It cannot be denied [this is just after he has quoted a passage of Taddeo with regard to dreams] that Taddeo's expressions have a certain liveliness all their own that gives us some idea why he was looked upon as so good a teacher, a teacher who, as we know now, also gave instruction by the bedside of patients." Pagel adds, "Taddeo's greatest merit and his highest significance in medical education consist in the fact that a great many (*zahlreiche*) physicians followed directly in his footsteps and were counted as his pupils. They were all men, as we know them, who as writers and practitioners of medicine succeeded in going far beyond the level of mediocrity in what they accomplished."

This was the teacher who most influenced young Mondino when he came to the University of Bologna, for it seems not unlikely that as a medical student he was actually the pupil of Taddeo, then in a vigorous old age. If not, he was at least brought under the direct influence of the teaching tradition created during more than thirty years by that wonderful old man. Knowing what we do of Taddeo it is not surprising that his pupil should have accomplished work that was to influence succeeding generations more than any other of that wonderful thirteenth century. Dr. Pilcher in the article on "The Mondino Myth," so often placed under contribution in this sketch, says that "It needs no great stretch of the imagination to picture somewhat of the effect that contact with such a man as Taddeo di Alderotto[15] might have, in molding the character of his young neighbor and pupil, the chemist's son, who a few years later, by his devotion to the study of human anatomy, was to re-establish the practical pursuit of study on the human cadaver as the common privilege of the skilled physician, and was to engrave his own name deeply on the records of medicine."

Under this worthy compatriot and contemporary of the great Florentines, Mondino was inspired to be the teacher that did so much for Bologna. Until recent years it has usually been the custom to give too much significance to the work of the men whose names stand out most prominently in the early history of departments of the intellectual life. Mondino's reputation has shared in this exaggerative tendency to some extent, hence the necessity for realizing what was accomplished before his time and the fact that he only stands as the culmination of a progressive period. Carlyle spoke of Dante as the man in whom "ten silent centuries found a voice." The centuries, however, were only silent because the moderns did not know how to listen to their message. We know now that every country in Europe had a great contributor to literature in the century before Dante. The Cid, the Arthur Legends, the Nibelungen, the Troubadours, naturally led up to Dante. He was only the culmination of a great period of literature. We know now that men had worked in art before Cimabue and Giotto, and had done impressive work that made for the progress of art. These names, however, have come to represent in many minds the sort of solitary phenomena that Dante has seemed sometimes even to scholars.

Because Mondino did such good work in medical teaching it is sometimes declared, even in rather serious histories, that he was the first to accomplish anything in his department, and that before his time there is a blank. Some historians, for instance, have insisted that Mondino was the first to do human dissections, and that he did at most but two or three. Only those who are unacquainted with the magnificent development of surgery that took place during the preceding century, the evidence for which is so abundantly given in modern historians of medicine and especially in Gurlt's great work on the history of surgery, from which we have quoted enough to give a good idea of the extent to which the movement went, are likely to accept any such declaration. There could not have been all that successful surgery without much dissection not only of animals but also of human bodies. The teaching of dissection was not regularly organized until Mondino's time, but it seems very clear that even he must have dissected many more bodies than the number usually attributed to him. Professor Lewis Stephen Pilcher of Brooklyn, who made a special study of Mondino traditions in Bologna itself, and collected some of the early editions of his books, feels so acutely the absurdity of the ordinarily accepted tradition in this matter, that he has written a paper on the subject bearing the suggestive title, "The Mondino Myth." He says:[16]

> "We are accustomed to think of the practice of dissection as having been re-created by

Mondino, and at once fully developed, springing into acceptance. The year 1315 is the generally accepted date for the first public anatomical demonstration upon a human body made by Mondino, and yet it is true that among the laws promulgated by Frederick II, more than seventy-five years before (A.D. 1231), was included a decree that a human body should be dissected at Salernum at least once in five years in the presence of the assembled physicians and surgeons of the kingdom, and that in the regulations established for admission to the practice of medicine and surgery in the kingdom it was decreed that no surgeon should be admitted to practise unless he should bring testimonials from the masters teaching in the medical faculty, that he was 'learned in the anatomy of human bodies, and had become perfect in that part of medicine without which neither incisions could safely be made nor fractures cured.'

"Salernum was notable in its legalization of the dissection of human bodies before the first public work of Mondino, for, according to a document of the Maggiore Consiglio of Venice of 1308, it appears that there was a college of medicine at Venice which was even then authorized to dissect a body every year. Common experience tells us that the embodiment of such regulations into formal law would occur only after a considerable preceding period of discussion, and in this particular field of clandestine practice. It is too much to ask us to believe that in all this period, from the date of the promulgation of Frederick's decree of 1231 to the first public demonstration by Mondino, at Bologna in 1315, the de cree had been a dead letter and no human body had been anatomized. It is true there is not, as far as I am aware, any record of any such work, and commentators and historians of a later date have, without exception, accepted the view that none was done, and thereby heightened the halo assigned to Mondino as the one who ushered in a new era. Such a view seems to me to be incredible. Be that as it may, it is undeniable that at the beginning of the 14th century the idea of dissecting the human body was not a novel one; the importance of a knowledge of the intimate structure of the body had already been appreciated by divers ruling bodies, and specific regulations prescribing its practice had been enacted. It is more reasonable to believe that in the era immediately preceding that of Mondino human bodies were being opened and after a fashion anatomized. All that we know of the work of Mondino suggests that it was not a new enterprise in which he was a pioneer, but rather that he brought to an old practice a new enthusiasm and better methods, which, caught on the rising wave of interest in medical teaching at Bologna, and preserved by his own energy as a writer in the first original systematic treatise written since the time of Galen, created for him in subsequent uncritical times the reputation of being the Restorer of the practice of anatomizing the human body, the first one to demonstrate and teach such knowledge since the time of the Ptolemaic anatomists, Erasistratus and Herophilus.

"The changes have been rung by medical historians upon a casual reference in

Mondino's chapter on the uterus to the bodies of two women and one sow which he had dissected, as if these were the first and the only cadavers dissected by him. The context involves no such construction. He is enforcing a statement that the size of the uterus may vary, and to illustrate it remarks that 'a woman whom I anatomized in the month of January last year, viz., 1315 Anno Christi, had a larger uterus than one whom I anatomized in the month of March of the same year.' And further, he says that 'the uterus of a sow which I dissected in 1316 (the year in which he was writing) was a hundred times greater than any I have seen in the human female, for she was pregnant and contained thirteen pigs.' These happen to be the only reference to specific bodies that he makes in his treatise. But it is a far cry to wring out of these references the conclusion that these are the only dissections he made. It is quite true that if we incline to enshroud his work in a cloud of mystery and to figure it as an unprecedented awe-inspiring feature to break down the prejudices of the ages, it is easy to think of him as having timidly profaned the human body by his anatomizing zeal in but one or two instances. His own language, however, throughout his book is that of a man who was familiar with the differing conditions of the organs found in many different bodies; a man who was habitually dissecting."

(Quotations from the work of Mundinus showing his familiarity with dissections. The leaf and line references are to the Dryander edition, Marburg, 1541.)

> "I do not consider separately the anatomy of component parts, because their anatomy does not appear clearly in the fresh subject, but rather in those macerated in water." (Leaf 2, lines 8-13.)
>
> "... these differences are more noticeable in the cooked or perfectly dried body, and so you need not be concerned about them, and perhaps I will make an anatomy upon such a one at another time and will write what I shall observe with my own senses, as I have proposed from the beginning." (Leaf 60, lines 14-17.)
>
> "What the members are to which these nerves come cannot well be seen in such a dissection as this, but it should be liquefied with rain water, and this is not contemplated in the present body." (Leaf 60, lines 31-33.)
>
> "After the veins you will note many muscles and many large and strong cords, the complete anatomy of which you will not endeavor to find in such a body but in a body dried in the sun for three years, as I have demonstrated at another time; I also declared completely their number, and wrote the anatomy of the muscles of the arms, hands, and feet in a lecture which I gave over the first, second, third, and fourth subjects." (Leaf 61, lines 1-7.)

Very probably the best evidence that we have of the comparative frequency at least of dissection at this time is to be found in the records of a trial for body-snatching that occurred in Bologna. The details would remind one very much of what we know of the difficulties with regard to dissection in America a couple of generations ago, when no bodies were provided by law for dissection purposes. In the course of some studies for the history of the New York State Medical Society (New York, 1906) I found that nearly every one of the first half dozen presidents of the New York Academy of Medicine, which is not much more than sixty years old, had had body-snatching experiences when they were younger. Dr. Samuel Francis, the medico-historical writer, tells of a personal expedition across the ferry in the winter time, bringing a body from a Long Island graveyard. In order to avoid the constables on the Long Island side and the police on the New York side, because there had been a number of cases of body-snatching recently and the authorities were on the lookout, the corpse was placed sitting beside the physician who drove the wagon, with a cloak wrapped around it, as if it were a living person specially protected against the cold. Similar experiences were not unusual. The lack of bodies for dissection is sometimes attributed to religious scruples, but they have very little to do with it, as at all times men have refused to allow the bodies of their friends to be treated as anatomical material. This is the natural feeling of abhorrence and not at all religious. It is only when there are many unclaimed bodies of strangers and the poor, as happens in large cities, that there can be an abundance of anatomical material.

The details of this body-snatching case are strangely familiar to those who know the history of similar cases before the middle of the nineteenth century. The case occurred in 1319 in Bologna, just four years after Mondino's public dissections. Four students were involved in the charge of body-snatching, all of them from outside the city of Bologna itself, three from Milan and one from Piacenza. In modern experience, too, as a rule, students from outside of the town where the medical college was situated, were always a little readier than natives to violate graveyards. These four students were accused of having gone at night to the Cemetery of St. Barnabas, outside the gate of San Felice,—suburban graveyards were usually the scene of such exploits,—and to have dug up the body of a certain criminal named Pasino, who had been hanged a few days before. They carried the body to the school in the Parish of San Salvatore, where Alberto Zancari was teaching. The resurrection had been accomplished without witnesses, but there were several witnesses who testified that they recognized the body of Pasino in the school and students occupied with its dissection. If evidence for the zeal of the medical students of that time for dissection were needed, surely we have it in the testimony at this trial. At a time when body-snatching has become a criminal offence usually there have been many repeated occurrences of it before the parties are brought to trial, so that it seems not unlikely that a good many dissections of illegally secured bodies were being done at Bologna at this time.

We know of a regulation of the University in force at this time, which required the teachers at the University to do an anatomy or dissection for students if they secured a body for that purpose. The students seem to have used all sorts of influence, political, monetary, diplomatic, and ecclesiastical, in order to secure the bodies of criminals. Sometimes when they failed in their purpose they waited until after burial and then took the body without leave. When we recall the awfully deterrent condition in which bodies must have been that were thus provided for dissecting purposes, it is easy to understand that the enthusiasm of the students for dissection must have been at a very high pitch. Certainly it was far higher than at the present day, when, in spite of the fact that our dissecting-rooms have very few of the old-time dangers and unpleasantnesses, dissection is only practised with assiduity if special care is exercised in requiring attendance and superintending the work of the department.

In my book on "The Popes and Science" I have gathered the traditions relating to Mondino's assistants in the chair of anatomy at Bologna. They furnish abundant evidence of the fact that dissections, far from being uncommon, must have been not at all infrequent at the north Italian universities at this time. Curiously enough, one of these assistants was a young woman who, as was not infrequently the custom at this time in the Italian universities, was matriculated as a student at Bologna. She took up first philosophy, and afterwards anatomy, under Mondino. While it is not generally realized, co-education was quite common at the Italian universities of the thirteenth and fourteenth centuries, and at no time since the foundation of the universities has a century passed in

Italy without distinguished women occupying professors' chairs at some of the Italian universities. This young woman, Alessandra Giliani, of Persiceto, a country district not far from Bologna, took up the study of anatomy with ardor and, strange as it may appear, became especially enthusiastic about dissection. She became so skilful that she was made the prosector of anatomy, that is, one who prepares bodies for demonstration by the professors.

According to the "Cronaca Persicetana," quoted by Medici in his "History of the Anatomical School at Bologna":

"She became most valuable to Mondino because she would cleanse most skilfully the smallest vein, the arteries, all ramifications of the vessels, without lacerating or dividing them, and to prepare them for demonstration she would fill them with various colored liquids, which, after having been driven into the vessels, would harden without destroying the vessels. Again, she would paint these same vessels to their minute branches so perfectly and color them so naturally that, added to the wonderful explanations and teachings of the master, they brought him great fame and credit." The whole passage shows a wonderful anticipation of our most modern methods—injection, painting, hardening—of making anatomical preparations for class and demonstration purposes.

Some of the details of the story have been doubted, but her memorial tablet, erected at the time of her death in the Church of San Pietro e Marcellino of the Hospital of Santa

Maria de Mareto, gives all the important facts, and tells the story of the grief of her fiancé, who was himself Mondino's other assistant.[17] This was Otto Agenius, who had made for himself a name as an assistant to the chair of anatomy in Bologna, and of whom there were great hopes entertained because he had already shown signs of genius as an investigator in anatomy. These hopes were destined to grievous disappointment, however, for Otto died suddenly, before he had reached his thirtieth year. The fact that both these assistants of Mondino died young and suddenly, would seem to point to the fact that probably dissection wounds in those early days proved even more fatal than they occasionally did a century or more ago, when the proper precautions against them were not so well understood. The death of Mondino's two prosectors in early years would seem to hint at some such unfortunate occurrence.

As regards the evidence of what the young man had accomplished before his untimely death, probably the following quotation, which Medici has taken from one of the old chroniclers, will give the best idea:

> "What advantage indeed might not Bologna have had from Otto Agenius Lustrulanus, whom Mondino had used as an assiduous prosector, if he had not been taken away by a swift and lamentable death before he had completed the sixth lustrum of his life!"

How well the tradition created by Mondino continued at the university will be best understood from what we know of Guy de Chauliac's visit to the medical school here about the middle of the century. The great French surgeon tells us that he came to Bologna to study anatomy under the direction of Mondino's successor, Bertruccius. When he wrote his preface to his great surgery he recalled this teaching of anatomy at Bologna and said, "It is necessary and useful to every physician to know, first of all, anatomy. For this purpose the study of books is indeed useful, but it is not sufficient to explain those things which can only be appreciated by the senses and which need to be seen in the dead body itself." He advises his students to consult Mundinus' treatise but to demonstrate its details for themselves on the dead body. He relates that he himself had often, *multitoties,* done this, especially under the direction of Bertruccius at Bologna. Curiously enough, as pointed out by Professor Pilcher, Mondino had used this same word *multitotiens* (the variant spelling makes no difference in the meaning) in speaking about his own work. In describing the hypogastric lesion he mentions that he had demonstrated certain veins in it many times, *multitotiens.*

Mondino was just past fifty when he finished his little book and permitted copies of it to be made. Though the book occurs so early in the history of modern book-making the author offers his excuses to the public for writing it, and quotes the authority of Galen, to whom he turns in other difficult situations, for justification. As prefaces go, Mondino's is so like that of many an author of more recent date that his words have a bibliographic, as well as a personal, interest. He said:

> "A work upon any science or art—as saith Galen—is issued for three reasons: first, that one may satisfy his friends. Second, that he may exercise his best mental powers. Third, that he may be saved from the oblivion incident to old age. Therefore, moved by these three causes, I have proposed to my pupils to compose a certain work on medicine.
>
> "And because a knowledge of the parts to be subjected to medicine (which is the human body, and the names of its various divisions) is a part of medical science, as saith Averrhoes in his first chapter, in the section on the definition of medicine, for this reason among others, I have set out to lay before you the knowledge of the parts of the human body which is derived from anatomy, not attempting to use a lofty style, but the rather that which is suitable to a manual of procedure."

Some of the early editions of Mondinus' book are said, according to old writers, to have contained illustrations. None of these copies have come down to us, but the assertion is made so definitely that it seems likely to have been the case. The editions that we have contain wood engravings of the method of making a dissection as frontispiece, so that it would not be difficult to think of further such illustrations having been employed in the book itself. As we note in the chapter on "Great Surgeons of the Medieval Universities," Mondeville, according to Guy de Chauliac, had pictures of anatomical preparations which he used for teaching purposes. It is easy to understand that the value of such aids would be recognized at a time when the difficulty of preserving bodies made it necessary to do dissections hurriedly so as to get the rapidly decomposing material out of the way. Beyond his book and certain circumstances connected with it we know very little about Mondino. What we know, however, enables us to conclude that, like many another great teacher, he must have had the special faculty of inspiring his students with an ardent enthusiasm for the work that they were taking under him. Hence the body-snatching and other stories. Mondino continued to be held in high estimation by the Bolognese for centuries after his death. Dr. Pilcher calls attention to the fact that his sepulchral tablet, which is in the portico of the Church of San Vitari in Bologna, and a replica of which he was allowed to have made in order to bring it to America, is the only one of the sepulchral tablets in the great churches of Florence, San Domenico, San Martino, the Cathedral and the Cloister of San Giacomo degli Ermitani, which has not been removed from its original location and placed in the halls of the Civic Museum. Their removal he considers "a kind of desecration which does violence to one's sense of sanctity and propriety." "Fortunately, thus far, the Mondino Tablet has escaped the spoiler." Very probably Dr. Pilcher's replica of the tablet which he was required to deposit in the Civic Museum at the time when the copy was made to be brought to America may save the tablet to be seen in its original position for many generations.

Mondino's career is of special interest because it foreshadows the life and accomplishment of many another maker of medicine of the after time. He did a great new thing in medicine in organizing regular public dissections, and then in making a manual that would facilitate the work. He waited patiently for years before completing his book in order that it might be the fruit of long experience, and so be more helpful to others. He was so modest as to require urging to secure the publication. He had the reward of his patience in the popularity of his little work for centuries after his time. The glimpse that we get of his relations to his young assistants, Agenius and Alessandra, seems to show us a teacher of distinct personal magnetism. Undoubtedly the reputation of his book did much for not only the medical school of the University of Bologna, but also for the medical schools of other north Italian universities, and helped to bring to them the crowds of students that flocked there during the fourteenth and fifteenth centuries.

Taddeo and Mondino turned the attention of the medical students of their generations Bolognawards. Before that time they had mainly gone to Salerno. After their time most of the ardent students of medicine felt that they must study for a time at least at Bologna. Other important medical schools of Italian universities at Padua, at Vicenza, at Piacenza, arose and prospered. During the time when the political troubles of Italy reached a climax about the middle of the fourteenth century, while the Popes were at Avignon, there was a remission in the attendance at all the Italian universities, but with the Popes' return to Rome and the coming of even comparative peace to Italy, Bologna once more became the term of medical pilgrimages for students from all over the world. In the meantime Mondino's book went forth to be the most used text-book of its kind until Vesalius' great work came to replace it. To have ruled in the world of anatomy for two centuries as the best known of teachers is of itself a distinction that shows us at once the teaching power and the scientific ability of this professor of anatomy of Bologna in the early fourteenth century.

X

GREAT SURGEONS OF THE MEDIEVAL UNIVERSITIES

Strange as it may appear to those who have not watched the development of our knowledge of the Middle Ages in recent years the most interesting feature in the medical departments and, indeed, of the post-graduate work generally of the medieval universities, is that in surgery. There is a very general impression that this department of medicine did not develop until quite recent years, and that particularly it failed to develop to any extent in the Middle Ages. A good many of the historians of this period, indeed, though never the special historians of medicine, have even gone far afield in order to find some reason why surgery did not develop at this time. They have insisted that the Church by its prohibition of the shedding of blood, first to monks and friars, and then to the secular clergy, prevented the normal development of surgery. Besides they add that Church opposition to anatomy completely precluded all possibility of any genuine natural evolution of surgery as a science.

There is probably no more amusing feature of quite a number of supposedly respectable and presumably authoritative historical works written in English than this assumption with regard to the absence of surgery during the later Middle Ages. Only the most complete ignorance of the actual history of medicine and surgery can account for it. The writers who make such assertions must never have opened an authoritative medical history. Nothing illustrates so well the expression of the editors of the "Cambridge Modern History" referred to more than once in these pages that "in view of changes and of gains such as these [the jointing of original documents] it has become impossible for historical writers of the present day to trust without reserve even to the most respected secondary authority. The honest student finds himself continually deserted, retarded, misled by the classics of historical literature." Fortunately for us this sweeping condemnation does not hold to any great extent for the medical historical classics. All of the classic historians of medicine tell us much of the surgery of the thirteenth and fourteenth centuries, and in recent years the republication of old texts and the further study of manuscript documents of various kinds have made it very clear that there is almost no period in the history of the world when surgery was so thoroughly and successfully cultivated as during the rise and development of the universities and their medical schools in the thirteenth and fourteenth centuries.

It is interesting to trace the succession of great contributors to surgery during these two centuries. We know their teaching not from tradition, but from their text-books so faithfully preserved for us by their devoted students, who must have begrudged no time and spared no labor in copying, for many of the books are large, yet exist in many manuscript copies.

Modern surgery may be said to owe its origin to a school of surgeons, the leaders of whom were educated at Salerno in the early part of the thirteenth century, and who, teaching at various north Italian universities, wrote out their surgical principles and experiences in a series of important contributions to that department of medical science. The fact that the origin of the school was at Salerno, where, as is well known, Arabian influence counted for much and for which Constantine's translations of Arabian works proved such a stimulus a century before, makes most students conclude that this later medieval surgical development is simply a continuation of the Arabian surgery that, as we have seen, developed very interestingly during the earlier Middle Ages. Any such idea, however, is not founded on the realities of the situation, but on an assumption with regard to the extent of Arabian influence. Gurlt in his "History of Surgery" (Vol. I, page 701) completely contradicts this idea, and says with regard to the first of the great Italian writers on surgery, Rogero, that "though Arabian works on surgery had been brought over to Italy by Constantine Africanus a hundred years before Roger's time, these exercised no influence over Italian surgery in the next century, and there is scarcely a trace of the surgical knowledge of the Arabs to be found in Roger's works."

It is in the history of medicine particularly that it is possible to trace the true influence of the Arabs on European thought in the later Middle Ages. We have already seen in the chapter on Salerno that Arabian influence did harm to Salernitan medical teaching. The school of Salerno itself had developed simple, dietetic, hygienic, and general remedial measures that included the use of only a comparatively small amount of drugs. Its teachers emphasized nature's curative powers. With Arabian influence came polypharmacy, distrust of nature, and attempts to cure disease rather than help nature. In surgery, which developed very wonderfully in the thirteenth and fourteenth centuries, Salerno must be credited with the incentive that led up to the marvellous development that came. With this, however, Arabian influence has nothing to do. Gurlt, besides calling attention to the fact that the author of the first great text-book on the subject not only did not draw his inspiration from Arab sources, insisted that "instead of any Arabisms being found in his [Roger's] writings many Græcisms occur." The Salernitan school of surgery drank at the fountain-head of Greek surgery. Apart from Greek sources Roger's book rests entirely upon his own experiences, those of his teachers and his colleagues, and the tradition in surgery that had developed at Salerno. This tradition was entirely from the Greek. Roger himself says in one place, "We have resolved to write out deliberately our methods of operation such as they have been derived from our own experience and that of our colleagues and illustrious men."

ROGER, ROLAND, AND THE FOUR MASTERS

Ruggero, or Rogero, who is also known as Rogerio and Rogerus with the adjective Parmensis, or Salernitanus, of Parma or of Salerno, and often in German and English history simply as Roger, lived at the end of the twelfth or the beginning of the thirteenth century and probably wrote his text-book about 1180. This text-book was, according to tradition, originally drafted for his lessons in surgery at Salerno. It attracted much attention and after being commented on by his pupil Rolando, the work of both of them being subsequently annotated by the Four Masters, this combined work became the basis of modern surgery. Roger was probably born either in Palermo or Parma. There are traditions of his having taught for a while at Paris and at the University of Montpellier, though these are not substantiated. His book was printed at Venice in 1546, and has been lately reprinted by De Renzi in his "Collectio Salernitana."

Roland was a pupil of Roger's, and the two names that often occur in medieval romance became associated in a great historic reality as a consequence of Roland's commentary on his master's work, which was a favorite text-book in surgery for a good while in the thirteenth century at Salerno. Some space will be given to the consideration of their surgical teaching after a few words with regard to some disciples who made a second commentary, adding to the value of the original work.

This is the well-known commentary of the Four Masters, a text-book of surgery written somewhat in the way that we now make text-books in various departments of medicine, that is, by asking men who have made specialties of certain subjects to write on that subject and then bind them all together in a single volume. It represents but another striking reminder that most of our methods are old, not new as we are likely to imagine them. The Four Masters took the works of Roger and Rolando, acknowledged their indebtedness much more completely than do our modern writers on all occasions, I fear, and added their commentaries.

Gurlt says ("Geschichte der Chirurgie," Vol. I, p. 703) that "in spite of the fact that there is some doubt about the names of the authors, this volume constitutes one of the most important sources for the history of surgery of the later Middle Ages and makes it very clear that these writers drew their opinions from a rich experience." It is rather easy to illustrate from the quotations given in Gurlt or from the accounts of their teaching in Daremberg or De Renzi some features of this experience that can scarcely fail to be surprising to modern surgeons. For instance, what is to be found in this old text-book of surgery with regard to fractures of the skull is likely to be very interesting to surgeons at all times. One might be tempted to say that fewer men would die every year in prison cells who ought to be in hospitals, if the old-time teaching was taken to heart. For there are rather emphatic directions not to conclude because the scalp is unwounded that there can be no fracture of the skull. Where nothing can be felt care must be exercised in getting the history of the case. For instance, if a man is hit by a metal instrument shaped like the clapper of a bell or by a heavy key, or by a rounded instrument made of lead—this would remind one very much of the lead pipe of the modern time, so fruitful of mistakes of diagnosis in head injuries—special care must be taken to look for symptoms in spite of the lack of an external penetrating wound. Where there is good reason to suspect a fracture because of the severity of the injury, the scalp should be incised and a fracture of the cranium looked for carefully. That is carrying the exploratory incision pretty far. If a fracture is found the surgeon should trephine so as to relieve the brain of any pressure of blood that might be affecting it.

There are many warnings, however, of the danger of opening the skull and of the necessity for definitely deciding beforehand that there is good reason for so doing. How carefully their observations had been made and how well they had taken advantage of their opportunities, which were, of course, very frequent in those warlike times when firearms were unknown, hand-to-hand conflict common, and blunt weapons were often used, can be appreciated very well from some of the directions. For instance, they knew of the possibility of fracture by *contrecoup*. They say that "quite frequently though the percussion comes in the anterior part of the cranium, the cranium is fractured on the opposite part."[18] They even seem to have known of accidents such as we now discuss in connection with the laceration of the middle meningeal artery. They warn surgeons of the possibilities of these cases. They tell the story of "a youth who had a very small wound made by a thrown stone and there seemed no serious results or bad signs. He died the next day, however. His cranium was opened and a large amount of black blood was found coagulated about his dura mater."

There are many interesting things said with regard to depressed fractures and the necessity for elevating the bone. If the depressed portion is wedged then an opening should be made with the trephine and an elevating instrument called a spatumen used to relieve the pressure. Great care should be taken, however, in carrying out this procedure lest the bone of the cranium itself, in being lifted, should injure the soft structures within. The dura mater should be carefully protected from injury as well as the pin. Care should especially be exercised at the brow and the rear of the head and at the commissures (*proram et pupim et commissuras*), since at these points the dura mater is likely to be adherent. Perhaps the most striking expression, the word *infect* being italicized by Gurlt, is: "In elevating the cranium be solicitous lest you should infect or injure the dura mater."

For wounds of the scalp sutures of silk are recommended because this resists putrefaction and holds the wound edges together. Interrupted sutures about a finger-breadth apart are recommended. "The lower part of the wound should be left open so that the cure may proceed properly." Red powder was strewed over the wound and the leaf of a plant set above it. In the lower angle of the wound a pledget of lint for drainage purposes was inlaid. Hemorrhage was prevented by pressure, by the binding on of *burnt* wool firmly, and by the ligature of veins and by the cautery.

There are rather interesting discussions of the prognosis of wounds of the head, especially such as may be determined from general symptoms in this commentary of the Four

Masters on Roger's and Rolando's treatises. If an acute febrile condition develops, the wound is mortal. If the patient loses the use of the hands and feet or if he loses his power of direction, or his sensation, the wound is mortal. If a universal paralysis comes on, the wound is mortal. For the treatment of all these wounds careful precautions are suggested. Cold was supposed to be particularly noxious to them. Operations on the head were not to be done in cold weather and, above all, not in cold places. The air where such operations were done must be warmed artificially. Hot plates should surround the patient's head while the operation was being performed. If this were not possible they were to be done by candlelight, the candle being held as close as possible in a warm room. These precautions are interesting as foreshadowing many ideas of much more modern time and especially indicating how old is the idea that cold may be taken in wounds. In popular medicine this still has its place. Whenever a wound does badly in the winter time patients are sure that they have taken cold. Such popular medical ideas are always derived from supposedly scientific medicine, and until we learned about microbes physicians used the same expressions. We have not got entirely away from them yet.

These old surgeons must have had many experiences with fractures at the base of the skull. Hemorrhages from the mouth and nose, for instance, and from the ears were considered bad signs. They were inclined to suggest that openings into the skull should be discovered by efforts to demonstrate a connection between the mouth and nares and the brain cavity. For instance, in their commentary the Four Masters said: "Let the patient hold his mouth and nostrils tight shut and blow strongly." If there was any lessening of the pressure or any appearance of air in the wound in the scalp, then a connection between the mouth and nose was diagnosticated. This is ingenious but eminently dangerous because of the infectious material contained in the nasal and oral cavities, so likely to be forced by such pressure into the skull. They were particularly anxious to detect linear fractures. One of their methods of negative diagnosis for fractures of the skull was that if the patient were able to bring his teeth together strongly, or to crack a nut without pain, then there was no fracture present. One of the commentators, however, adds to this "*sed hoc aliquando fallit*—but this sign sometimes fails." Split or crack fractures were also diagnosticated by the method suggested by Hippocrates of pouring some colored fluid over the skull after the bone was exposed, when the linear fracture would show by coloration. The Four Masters suggest a sort of red ink for this purpose.

While they have so much to say about fractures of the skull and insist, over and over again, that though all depressed fractures need treatment and many fissure fractures require trepanation, still great care must be exercised in the selection of cases. They say, for instance, that surgeons who in every serious wound of the head have recourse to the trephine must be looked upon as "fools and idiots" (*idioti et stolidi*). In the light of what we now know about the necessity for absolute cleanliness,—asepsis as we have come to call it,—it is rather startling to note the directions that are given to a surgeon to be observed on the day when he is to do a trepanation. For obvious reasons I prefer to quote it in the Latin: "*Et nota quod die ilia cavendum est medico a coitu et malis cibis aera corrumpentibus, ut sunt allia, cepe, et hujusmodi, et colloquio mulieris menstruosæ, et manus ejus debent esse mundæ, etc.*" My quotation is from Gurlt, Vol. I, p. 707. The directions are most interesting. The surgeon's hands must be clean, he must avoid the taking of food that may corrupt the air, such as onions, leeks, and the like; must avoid menstruating and other women, and in general must keep himself in a state of absolute cleanliness.

To read a passage like this separated from its context and without knowing anything about the wonderful powers of observation of the men from whom it comes, it would be very easy to think that it is merely a set of general directions which they had made on some general principle, perhaps quite foolish in itself. We know, however, that these men had by observation detected nearly every feature of importance in fractures of the skull, their indications and contra-indications for operation and their prognosis. They had anticipated nearly everything of importance that has come to be insisted on even in our own time in the handling of these difficult cases. It is not unlikely, therefore, that they had also arrived at the recognition by observations on many patients that the satisfactory after-course of these cases which were operated on by the surgeon after due regard to such meticulous cleanliness as is suggested in the paragraph I have quoted, made it very clear that these aseptic precautions, as we would call them, were extremely important for the outcome of the case and, therefore, were well worth the surgeon's attention, though they must have required very careful precautions and considerable self-denial. Indeed this whole subject, the virtual anticipation of our nineteenth-century principles of aseptic surgery in the thirteenth century, is not a dream nor a far-fetched explanation when one knows enough about the directions that were laid down in the surgical text-books of that time.

THE NORTH ITALIAN SURGEONS

After Roger and Rolando and the Four Masters, who owe the inspiration for their work to Salerno and the south of Italy, comes a group of north Italian surgeons: Bruno da Longoburgo, usually called simply Bruno; Theodoric and his father, Hugo of Lucca, and William of Salicet. Immediately following them come two names that belong, one almost feels, to a more modern period: Mondino, the author of the first text-book on dissection, and Lanfranc (the disciple of William of Salicet), who taught at Paris and "gave that primacy to French surgery which it maintained all the centuries down to the nineteenth" (Pagel). It might very well be thought that this group of Italian surgeons had very little in their writings that would be of any more than antiquarian interest for the modern time. It needs but a little knowledge of their writings as they have come down to us to show how utterly false any such opinion is. To Hugo da Lucca and his son Theodoric we owe the introduction and the gradual bringing into practical use of various methods of anæsthesia. They used opium and mandragora for this purpose and later employed an inhalant mixture, the composition of which is not absolutely known. They seem, however, to have been very successful in producing insensibility to pain for even rather serious and complicated and somewhat lengthy operations. Indeed it is to this that must be attributed most of their surprising success as surgeons at this early date.

We are so accustomed to think that anæsthesia was discovered about the middle of the nineteenth century in America that we forget that literature is full of references in Tom Middleton's (seventeenth century) phrase to "the mercies of old surgeons who put their patients to sleep before they cut them." Anæsthetics were experimented with almost as zealously, during the latter half of the thirteenth century at least, as during the latter half of the nineteenth century. They were probably not as successful as we are, but they did succeed in producing insensibility to pain, otherwise they could never have operated to the extent they did. Moreover the traditions show that the Da Luccas particularly had invented a method that left very little to be desired in this matter of anæsthesia. A reference to the sketch of Guy de Chauliac in this volume will show how practical the method was in his time.

Nearly the same story as with regard to anæsthetics has to be repeated for what are deemed so surely modern developments,—asepsis and antisepsis. I have already suggested that Roger seems to have known how extremely important it was to approach operations upon the skull with the most absolute cleanliness. There are many hints of the same kind in other writers which show that this was no mere accidental remark, but was a definite conclusion derived from experience and careful observation of results. We find much more with regard to this same subject in the writings of the group of northern Italian surgeons and especially in the group of those associated with William of Salicet. Professor Clifford Allbutt, Regius Professor of Medicine at the University of Cambridge, England, in his address before the St. Louis World's Fair Congress of Arts and Science in 1904, did not hesitate to declare that William discussed the causes for union by first intention and the modes by which it might be obtained. He, too, insisted on cleanliness as the most important factor in having good surgical results, and all of this group of men, in operating upon septic cases, used stronger wine as a dressing. This exerted, as will be readily understood, a very definite antiseptic quality.

Evidently some details of the teaching of this group of great surgeons in northern Italy in the second half of the thirteenth century will make clearer to us how much the rising universities of the time were accomplishing in medicine and surgery as well as in their other departments. The dates of the origin of some of these universities should perhaps be recalled so as to remind readers how closely related they are to this great group of surgical teachers. Salerno was founded very early, probably in the tenth century, Bologna, Reggio, and Modena came into existence toward the end of the twelfth century; Vicenza, Padua, Naples, Vercelli, and Piacenza, as well as Arezzo, during the first half of the thirteenth century; Rome, Perugia, Trevizo, Pisa, Florence, Sienna, Lucca, Pavia, and Ferrara during the next century. The thirteenth century was the special flourishing period of the universities, and the medical departments, far from being behind, were leaders in accomplishment. (See my "The Thirteenth Greatest of Centuries," N. Y., 1908.)

BRUNO DA LONGOBURGO

The first of this important group of north Italian surgeons who taught at these universities was Bruno of Longoburgo. While he was born in Calabria, and probably studied in Salerno, his work was done at Vicenza, Padua, and Verona. His text-book, the "Chirurgia Magna," dedicated to his friend Andrew of Piacenza, was completed at Padua in January, 1252. Gurlt notes that he is the first of the Italian surgeons who quotes, besides the Greeks, the Arabian writers on surgery. Eclecticism had definitely come into vogue to replace exclusive devotion to the Greek authors, and men were taking what was good wherever they found it. Gurlt tells us that Bruno owed much of what he wrote to his own experience and observation. He begins his work by a definition of surgery, *chirurgia,* tracing it to the Greek and emphasizing that it means handwork. He then declares that it is the last instrument of medicine to be used only when the other two instruments,diet and potions, have failed. He insists that surgeons must learn by seeing surgical operations and watching them long and diligently. They must be neither rash nor over bold and should be extremely cautious about operating. While he says that he does not object to a surgeon taking a glass of wine, the followers of this specialty must not drink to such an extent as to disturb their command over themselves, and they must not be habitual drinkers. While all that is necessary for their art cannot be learned out of books, they must not despise books however, for many things can be learned readily from books, even about the most difficult parts of surgery. Three things the surgeon has to do: — "to bring together separated parts, to separate those that have become abnormally united, and to extirpate what is superfluous."

In his second chapter on healing he talks about healing by first and second intention. Wounds must be more carefully looked to in summer than in winter, because *putrefactio est major in aestate quam in hyeme,* putrefaction is greater in summer than in winter. For proper union care must be exercised to bring the wound edges accurately together and not allow hair, or oil, or dressings to come between them. In large wounds he considers stitching indispensable, and recommends for this a fine, square needle. The preferable suture material in his experience was silk or linen.

The end of the wound was to remain open in order that lint might be placed therein in order to draw off any objectionable material. He is particularly insistent on the necessity for drainage. In deep wounds special provision must be made, and in wounds of extremities the limb must be so placed as to encourage drainage. If drainage does not take place, then either the wound must be thoroughly opened, or if necessary a counter opening must be made to provide drainage. All his treatment of wounds is dry, however. Water, he considered, always did harm. We can readily understand that the water generally available and especially as surgeons saw it in camps and on the battlefield, was likely to do much more harm than good. In penetrating wounds of the belly cavity, if there was difficulty in bringing about the reposition of the intestines, they were first to be pressed back with a sponge soaked in warm wine. Other manipulations are suggested, and if necessary the wound must be enlarged. If the omentum finds its way out of the wound, all of it that is black or green must be cut off. In cases where the intestines are wounded they are to be sewed with a small needle and a silk thread and care is to be exercised in bringing about complete closure of the wound. This much will give a good idea of Bruno's thoroughness. Altogether, Gurlt, in his "History of Surgery," gives about fifteen large octavo pages of rather small type to a *brief* compendium of Bruno's teachings.

One or two other remarks of Bruno are rather interesting in the light of modern developments in medicine. For instance, he suggests the possibility of being able to feel a stone in the bladder by means of bimanual palpation. He teaches that mothers may often be able to cure hernias, both umbilical and inguinal, in children by promptly taking up the treatment of them as soon as noticed, bringing the edges of the hernial opening together by bandages and then preventing the reopening of the hernia by prohibiting wrestling and loud crying and violent motion. He has seen overgrowth of the mamma in men, and declares that it is due to nothing else but fat, as a rule. He suggests if it should hang down and be in the way on account of its size it should be extirpated. He seems to have known considerable about the lipomas and advises that they need only be removed in case they become bothersomely large. The removal is easy, and any bleeding that takes place may be stopped by means of the cautery. He divides rectal fistulæ into penetrating and non-penetrating, and suggests salves for the non-penetrating and the actual cautery for those that penetrate. He warns against the possibility of producing incontinence by the incision of deep fistulæ, for this would leave the patient in a worse state than before.

HUGH OF LUCCA

Bruno brought up with him the methods and principles of surgery from the south of Italy, but there seems to have been already in the north at least one distinguished surgeon who had made his mark. This was Ugo da Lucca or Ugo Luccanus, sometimes known in the modern times in German histories of medicine as Hugo da Lucca and in English, Hugh of Lucca. He flourished early in the thirteenth century. In 1214 he was called to Bologna to become the city physician, and joined the Bolognese volunteers in the crusade in 1218, being present at the siege of Damietta. He returned to Bologna in 1221 and was given the post of legal physician to the city. The civic statutes of Bologna are, according to Gurlt, the oldest monument of legal medicine in the Middle Ages. Ugo died not long after the middle of the century, and is said to have been nearly one hundred years old. Of his five sons, three became physicians. The most celebrated of these was Theodoric, who wrote a text-book of surgery in which are set down the traditions of surgery that had been practised in his father's life. Theodoric is especially enthusiastic in praise of his father, because he succeeded in bringing about such perfect healing of wounds with only wine and water and the ligature and without the employment of any ointments.

Ugo seems to have occupied himself much with chemistry. To him we owe a series of discoveries with regard to anodyne and anæsthetizing drugs. He is said to have been the first who taught the sublimation of arsenic. Unfortunately he left no writings after him, and all that we know of him we owe to the filial devotion of his son Theodoric.

THEODORIC

This son, after having completed his medical studies at the age of about twenty-three, entered the Dominican Order, then only recently established, but continued his practice of medicine undisturbed. His ecclesiastical preferment was rapid. He attracted the attention of the Bishop of Valencia, and became his chaplain in Rome. At the age of about fifty he was made a bishop in South Italy and later transferred to the Bishopric of Cervia, not far from Ravenna. Most of his life seems to have been passed in Bologna however, and he continued to practise medicine, devoting his fees, however, entirely to charity. His text-book of surgery was written about 1266 and is signed with his full name and title as Bishop of Cervia. Even at this time however, he still retained the custom of designating himself as a member of the Dominican Order.

The most interesting thing in the first book of his surgery is undoubtedly his declaration that all wounds should be treated only with wine and bandaging. Wine he insists on as the best possible dressing for wounds. It was the most readily available antiseptic that they had at that time, and undoubtedly both his father's recommendation of it and his own favorable experience with it were due to this quality. It must have acted as an excellent inhibitive agent of many of the simple forms of pus formation. At the conclusion of this first book he emphasizes that it is extremely important for the healing of wounds that the patient should have good blood, and this can only be obtained from suitable nutrition. It is essential therefore for the physician to be familiar with the foods which produce good blood in order that his wounded patients may be fed appropriately. He suggests, then, a number of articles of diet which are particularly useful in producing such a favorable state of the tissues as will bring about the rebirth of flesh and the adhesion of wound surfaces. Shortly before he emphasizes the necessity for not injuring nerves, though if nerves have been cut they should be brought together as carefully as possible, the wound edges being then approximated.

Probably the most interesting feature for our generation of the great text-books of the surgeons of the medieval universities is the occurrence in them of definite directions for securing union in surgical wounds, at least by first intention and their insistence on keeping wounds clear. The expression union by first intention comes to us from the olden time. They even boasted that the scars left after their incisions were often so small as to be scarcely noticeable. Such expressions of course could only have come from men who had succeeded in solving some of the problems of antisepsis that were solved once more in the generation preceding our own. With regard to their treatment of wounds, Professor Clifford Allbutt says:[19]

> "They washed the wound with wine, scrupulously removing every foreign particle; then they brought the edges together, not allowing wine nor anything else to remain within—dry adhesive surfaces were their desire. Nature, they said, produces the means of union in a viscous exudation, or natural balm, as it was afterwards called by Paracelsus, Paré, and Wurtz. In older wounds they did their best to obtain union by cleansing, desiccation, and refreshing of the edges. Upon the outer surface they laid only lint steeped in wine. Powders they regarded as too desiccating, for powder shuts in decomposing matters wine after washing, purifying, and drying the raw surfaces evaporates."

Theodoric comes nearest to us of all these old surgeons. The surgeon who in 1266 wrote: "For it is not necessary, as Roger and Roland have written, as many of their disciples teach, and as all *modern* surgeons profess, that pus should be generated in wounds. No error can be greater than this. Such a practice is indeed to hinder nature, to prolong the disease, and to prevent the conglutination and consolidation of the wound" was more than half a millennium ahead of his time. The italics in the word modern are mine, but might well have been used by some early advocate of antisepsis or even by Lord Lister himself.

Just six centuries almost to the year would separate the two declarations, yet they would be just as true at one time as at another. When we learn that Theodoric was proud of the beautiful cicatrices which he obtained without the use of any ointment, *pulcherrimas cicatrices sine unguento aliquo inducebat,* then further that he impugned the use of poultices and of oils on wounds, while powders were too drying and besides had a tendency to prevent drainage, the literal meaning of the Latin words *saniem incarcerare* is to "incarcerate sanious material," it is easy to understand that the claim that antiseptic surgery was anticipated six centuries ago is no exaggeration and no far-fetched explanation with modern ideas in mind of certain clever modes of dressing hit upon accidentally by medieval surgeons.

Theodoric's treatment of many practical problems is interesting for the modern time. For instance, in his discussion of cancer he says that there are two forms of the affection. One of them is due to a melancholy humor, a constitutional tendency as it were, and occurs especially in the breasts of women or latent in the womb. This is difficult of treatment and usually fatal. The other class consists of a deep ulcer with undermined edges, occurring particularly on the legs, difficult to cure and ready of relapse, but for which the outlook is not so bad. His description of *noli me tangere* and of lupus is rather practical. Lupus is "eating herpes," occurs mainly on the nose, or around the mouth, slowly increases, and either follows a preceding erysipelas or comes from some internal cause. *Noli me tangere* is a corroding ulcer, so called perhaps because irritation of it causes it to spread more rapidly. He thinks that deep cauterization of it is the best treatment. Since these are in the department of skin diseases this seems the place to mention that Theodoric describes salivation as occurring after the use of mercury for certain skin diseases. He has already shown that he knows of certain genital ulcers and sores on the genital regions and of distinctions between them.

WILLIAM OF SALICET

The third of the great surgeons in northern Italy was William of Salicet. He was a pupil of Bruno's and the master of Lanfranc. The first part of his life was passed at Bologna and the latter part as the municipal and hospital physician of Verona. He probably died about 1280. He was a physician as well as a surgeon and was one of those who insisted that the two modes of practising medicine should not be separated, or if they were both medicine and surgery would suffer. He thought that the physician learned much by seeing the interior of the body during life, while the surgeon was more conservative if he were a physician. It is curiously interesting to find that the Regius Professors at both Oxford and Cambridge in our time have expressed themselves somewhat similarly. Professor Clifford Allbutt is quite emphatic in this matter and Professor Osler is on record to the same effect. Following

Theodoric, William of Salicet did much to get away from the Arabic abuse of the cautery and brought the knife back to its proper place again as the ideal surgical instrument. Unlike those who had written before him, William quoted very little from preceding writers. Whenever he quotes his contemporaries it is in order to criticise them. He depended on his own experience and considered that it was only what he had actually learned from experience that he should publish for the benefit of others.

A very good idea of the sort of surgery that William of Salicet practised may be obtained even from the beginning of the first chapter of his first book. This is all with regard to surgery of the head. He begins with the treatment of hydrocephalus or, as he calls it, "water collected in the heads of children newly born." He rejects opening of the head by an incision because of the danger of it. In a number of cases, however, he had had success by puncturing the scalp and membranes with a cautery, though but a very small opening was made and the fluid was allowed to escape only drop by drop. He then takes up eye diseases, a department of surgery rather well developed at that time, as can be seen from our account of the work of Pope John XXI as an ophthalmologist during the thirteenth century. See *Ophthalmology* (January, 1909), reprinted in "Catholic Churchmen in Science," Philadelphia, The Dolphin Press, 1909.

William devotes six chapters to the diseases of the eyes and the eyelids. Then there are two chapters on affections of the ears. Foreign bodies and an accumulation of ear wax are removed by means of instruments. A polyp is either cut off or its pedicle bound with a ligature, and it is allowed to shrivel. The next chapter is on the nose. Nasal polyps were to be grasped with a sharp tenaculum, *cum tenacillis acutis,* and either wholly or partially extracted. Ranula was treated by being lifted well forward by means of a sharp iron hook and then split with a razor. It is evident that the tendency of these to fill up again was recognized, and accordingly it was recommended that vitriol powder, or alum with salt, be placed in the cavity for a time after evacuation in order to produce adhesive inflammation.

In the same chapter on the mouth one finds that William did not hesitate to perform what cannot but be considered rather extensive operations within the oral cavity. For instance, he tells of removing a large epulis and gives an account in detail of the case. To quote his own words: "I cured a certain woman from Piacenza who was suffering from fleshy tumor on the gums of the upper jaw, the tumor having grown to such a size above the teeth and the gums that it was as large or perhaps larger than a hen's egg. I removed it at four operations by means of heated iron instruments. At the last operation I removed the teeth that were loose with certain parts of the jawbone."

In the next chapter there is an account of the treatment of a remarkable case of abscess of the uvula. In the following chapter the swelling of cervical glands is taken up. In his experience expectant treatment of these was best. He advises internal medication with the building up of the general health, or suggests allowing the inflamed glands to empty themselves after pustulation. After much meddlesome surgery we are almost back to his methods again. He did not hesitate to treat goitre surgically, though he considered there were certain internal remedies that would benefit it. In obstinate cases he suggests the complete extirpation of cystic goitre, but if the sac is allowed to remain it should be thoroughly rubbed over on the inside with green ointment. He warns about the necessity for avoiding the veins and arteries in this operation, and says that "in this affection many large veins make their appearance and they find their way everywhere through the fleshy mass."

What I have given here is to be found in a little more than half a page of Gurlt's abstract of the first twenty chapters of Salicet's first book. Altogether Gurlt has more than ten pages of rather small print with regard to William; most of it is as interesting and as practical and as representative of anticipations of what is done in the modern time as what I have here quoted. William, as I have said, depended much more upon his own experience than upon what was to be found in text-books. He knew the old text-books very well however, but as a rule did not quote from them unless he had tried the recommendations for himself, or unless similar cases to these mentioned had come under his own observation. He was evidently a thoroughly observant physician, a skilled surgeon who was practical enough to see the simplest way to do things, and he proceeded to do them. It is no wonder that he influenced succeeding generations so much, nor that his great pupil, Lanfranc, continuing his tradition, founded a school of surgery in Paris, the influence of which was to endure almost down to our time, and give France a primacy in surgery until the nineteenth century.

LANFRANC

After Salicet's lifetime the focus of interest in surgery changes from Italy to France, and what is still more complimentary to William, it is through a favorite disciple of his that the change takes place. This was Lanfranchi, or Lanfranco, sometimes spoken of as Alanfrancus, who practised as physician and surgeon in Milan until banished from there by Matteo Visconti about 1290. He then went to Lyons, where in the course of his practice he attracted so much attention that he was offered the opportunity to teach surgery in Paris. He attracted what Gurlt calls an almost incredible number of scholars to his lessons in Paris, and by hundreds they accompanied him to the bedside of his patients and attended his operations. The dean of the medical faculty, Jean de Passavant, urged him to write a text-book of surgery, not only for the benefit of his students at Paris but for the sake of the prestige which this would confer on the medical school. Deans still urge the same reasons for writing. Lanfranc completed his surgery, called "Chirurgia Magna," in 1296, and dedicated it to Philippe le Bel, the then reigning French King. Ten years later he died, but in the meantime he had transferred Italian prestige in surgery from Italy to France and laid the foundations in Paris of a thoroughly scientific as well as a practical surgery, though this department of the medical school had been in a sadly backward state when he came.

In the second chapter of this text-book, the first containing the definition of surgery and general introduction, Lanfranc describes the qualities that in his opinion a surgeon should possess. He says, "It is necessary that a surgeon should have a temperate and moderate disposition. That he should have well-formed hands, long slender fingers, a strong body, not inclined to tremble and with all his members trained to the capable fulfilment of the wishes of his mind. He should be of deep intelligence and of a simple, humble, brave, but not audacious disposition. He should be well grounded in natural science, and should know not only medicine but every part of philosophy; should know logic well, so as to be able to understand what is written, to talk properly, and to support what he has to say by good reasons." He suggests that it would be well for the surgeon to have spent some time teaching grammar and dialectics and rhetoric, especially if he is to teach others in surgery, for this practice will add greatly to his teaching power. Some of his expressions might well be repeated to young surgeons in the modern time. "The surgeon should not love difficult cases and should not allow himself to be tempted to undertake those that are desperate. He should help the poor as far as he can, but he should not hesitate to ask for good fees from the rich."

Many generations since Lanfranc's time have used the word nerves for tendons. Lanfranc, however, made no such mistake. He says that the wounds of nerves, since the nerve is an instrument of sense and motion, are, on account of the greater sensitiveness which these structures possess, likely to involve much pain. Wounds along the length of the nerves are less dangerous than those across them. When a nerve is completely divided by a cross wound Lanfranc is of the opinion, though Theodoric and some others are opposed to it, that the nerve ends should be stitched together. He says that this suture insures the redintegration of the nerve much better. After this operation the restoration of the usefulness of the member is more complete and assured.

His description of the treatment of the bite of a rabid dog is interesting. A large cupping glass should be applied over the wound so as to draw out as much blood as possible. After this the wound should be dilated and thoroughly cauterized to its depths with a hot iron. It should then be covered with various substances that were supposed to draw, in order as far as possible to remove the poison. His description of how one may recognize a rabid animal is rather striking in the light of our present knowledge, for he seems to have realized that the main diagnostic element is a change in the disposition of the animal, but above all a definite tendency to lack playfulness. Lanfranc had seen a number of cases of true rabies, and describes and suggests treatment for them, though evidently without very much confidence in the success of the treatment.

The treatment of snake bites and the bites of other poisonous animals was supposed to follow the principles laid down for the bite of a mad dog, especially as regards the encouragement of free bleeding and the use of the cautery.

Lanfranc has many other expressions that one is tempted to quote, because they show a thinking surgeon of the old time, anticipating many supposedly modern ideas and conclusions. He is a particular favorite of Gurlt's, who has more than twenty-five large octavo, closely printed pages with regard to him. There is scarcely any development in our modern surgery that Lanfranc has not at least a hint of, certainly nothing in the surgery of a generation ago that does not find a mention in his book. On most subjects he has practical observations from his own experience to add to what was in surgical literature before his time. He quotes altogether more than a score of writers on surgery who had preceded him and evidently was thoroughly familiar with general surgical literature. There is scarcely an important surgical topic on which Gurlt does not find some interesting and personal remarks made by Lanfranc. All that we can do here is refer those who are interested in Lanfranc to his own works or Gurlt.

MONDEVILLE

The next of the important surgeons who were to bring such distinction to French surgery for five centuries was Henri de Mondeville. Writers usually quote him as Henricus. His latter name is only the place of his birth, which was probably not far from Caen in Normandy. It is spelled in so many different ways, however, by different writers that it is well to realize that almost anything that looks like Mondeville probably refers to him. Such variants as Mundeville, Hermondaville, Amondaville, Amundaville, Amandaville, Mandeville, Armandaville, Armendaville, Amandavilla occur. We owe a large amount of our information with regard to him to Professor Pagel, who issued the first edition of his book ever published (Berlin, 1892). It may seem surprising that Mondeville's work should have been left thus long without publication, but unfortunately he did not live long enough to finish it. He was one of the victims that tuberculosis claimed among physicians in the midst of their work. Though there are a great number of manuscript copies of his book, somehow Renaissance interest in it in its incompleted state was never aroused sufficiently to bring about a printed edition. Certainly it was not because of any lack of interest on the part of his contemporaries or any lack of significance in the work itself, for its printing has been one of the surprises afforded us in the modern time as showing how thoroughly a great writer on surgery did his work at the beginning of the fourteenth century.Gurlt, in his "History of Surgery," has given over forty pages, much of it small type, with regard to Mondeville, because of the special interest there is in his writing.[20]

His life is of particular interest for other reasons besides his subsequent success as a surgeon. He was another of the university men of this time who wandered far for opportunities in education. Though born in the north of France and receiving his preliminary education there, he made his medical studies towards the end of the thirteenth century under Theodoric in Italy. Afterwards he studied medicine in Montpellier and surgery in Paris. Later he gave at least one course of lectures at Montpellier himself and a series of lectures in Paris, attracting to both universities during his professorship a crowd of students from every part of Europe. One of his teachers at Paris had been his compatriot, Jean Pitard, the surgeon of Philippe le Bel, of whom he speaks as "most skilful and expert in the art of surgery," and it was doubtless to Pitard's friendship that he owed his appointment as one of the four surgeons and three physicians who accompanied the King into Flanders.

Besides his lectures, Mondeville had a large consultant practice and also had to accompany the King on his campaigns. This made it extremely difficult for him to keep continuously at the writing of his book. It was delayed in spite of his good intentions, and we have the picture that is so familiar in the modern time of a busy man trying to steal or make time for his writing. Unfortunately, in addition to other obstacles, Mondeville showed probably before he was forty the first symptoms of a serious pulmonary disease, presumably tuberculosis. He bravely fought it and went on with his work. As his end approached he sketched in lightly what he had hoped to treat much more formally, and then turned to what was to have been the last chapter of his book, the Antidotarium or suggestions of practical remedies against diseases of various kinds because his students and physician friends were urging him to complete this portion for them. We of the modern time are much less interested in that than we would have been in some of the portions of the work that Mondeville neglected in order to provide therapeutic hints for his disciples. But then the students and young physicians have always clamored for the practical—which so far at least in medical history has always proved of only passing interest.

It is often said that at this time surgery was mainly in the hands of barbers and the ignorant. Henri de Mondeville, however, is a striking example in contradiction of this. He must have had a fine preliminary education and his book shows very wide reading. There is almost no one of any importance who seriously touched upon medicine or surgery before his time whom Mondeville does not quote. Hippocrates, Aristotle, Dioscorides, Pliny, Galen, Rhazes, Ali Abbas, Abulcasis, Avicenna, Constantine Africanus, Averroës, Maimonides, Albertus Magnus, Hugo of Lucca, Theodoric, William of Salicet, Lanfranc are all quoted, and not once or twice but many times. Besides he has quotations from the poets and philosophers, Cato, Diogenes, Horace, Ovid, Plato, Seneca, and others. He was a learned man, devoting himself to surgery.

It is no wonder, then, that he thought that a surgeon should be a scholar, and that he needed to know much more than a physician. One of his characteristic passages is that in which he declares "it is impossible that a surgeon should be expert who does not know not only the principles, but everything worth while knowing about medicine," and then he added, "just as it is impossible for a man to be a good physician who is entirely ignorant of the art of surgery." He says further: "This our art of surgery, which is the third part of medicine (the other two parts were diet and drugs), is, with all due reverence to physicians, considered by us surgeons ourselves and by the non-medical as a more certain, nobler, securer, more perfect, more necessary, and more lucrative art than the other parts of medicine." Surgeons have always been prone to glory in their specialty.

Mondeville had a high idea of the training that a surgeon should possess. He says: "A surgeon who wishes to operate regularly ought first for a long time to frequent places in which skilled surgeons operate often, and he ought to pay careful attention to their operations and commit their technique to memory. Then he ought to associate himself with them in doing operations. A man cannot be a good surgeon unless he knows both the art and science of medicine and especially anatomy. The characteristics of a good surgeon are that he should be moderately bold, not given to disputations before those who do not know medicine, operate with foresight and wisdom, not beginning dangerous operations until he has provided himself with everything necessary for lessening the danger. He should have well-shaped members, especially hands with long, slender fingers, mobile and not tremulous, and with all his members strong and healthy so that he may perform all the good operations without disturbance of mind. He must be highly moral, should care for the poor for God's sake, see that he makes himself well paid by the rich, should comfort his patients by pleasant discourse, and should always accede to their requests if these do not interfere with the cure of the disease." "It follows from this," he says, "that the perfect surgeon is more than the perfect physician, and that while he must know medicine he must in addition know his handicraft."

Thinking thus, it is no wonder that he places his book under as noble patronage as possible. He says in the preface that he "began to write it for the honor and praise of Christ Jesus, of the Virgin Mary, of the Saints and Martyrs, Cosmas and Damian, and of King Philip of France as well as his four children, and on the proposal and request of Master William of Briscia, distinguished professor in the science of medicine and formerly physician to Pope Boniface IV and Benedict and Clement, the present Pope." His first book on anatomy he proposed to found on that of Avicenna and "on his personal experience as he has seen it." The second tractate on the treatments of wounds, contusions, and ulcers was founded on the second book of Theodoric "with whatever by recent study has been newly acquired and brought to light through the experience of modern physicians." He then confesses his obligations to his great master, John Pitard, and adds that all the experience that he has gained while operating, studying, and lecturing for many years on surgery will be made use of in order to enhance the value of the work. He hopes, however, to accomplish all this "briefly, quietly, and above all, charitably." There are many things in the preface that show us the reason for Mondeville's popularity, for they exhibit him as very sympathetically human in his interests.

While Mondeville is devoted to the principle that authority is of great value, he said that there was nothing perfect in things human, and successive generations of younger men often made important additions to what their ancestors had left them. While his work is largely a compilation, nearly everywhere it shows signs of the modification of his predecessors' opinions by the results of his own experience. His method of writing is, as Pagel declares, "always interesting, lively, and often full of meat." He had a teacher's instinct, for in several of the earlier manuscripts his special teaching is put in larger letters in order to attract students' attention.... He seems to have introduced or re-introduced into practice the idea of the use of a large magnet in order to extract portions of iron from the tissues. He made several modifications in needles and thread holders and invented a kind of small derrick for the extraction of arrows with barbs. Besides, he suggested the surrounding of the barbs of the arrows with tubes, to facilitate extraction. In his treatment of wounds, Pagel considers that as a writer and teacher he is far ahead of his predecessors and even of those who came after him in immediately subsequent generations. One of his great merits undoubtedly is that Guy de Chauliac, the father of modern surgery, in his text-book turned to him with a confidence that proclaims his admiration and how much he felt that he had gained from him.

One of the most interesting features of Mondeville's work is his insistence on the influence of the mind on the body and the importance of using this influence to the best advantage. It is especially important in Mondeville's opinion to keep a surgical patient from being moody. "Let the surgeon," says he, "take care to regulate the whole regimen of the patient's life for joy and happiness by promising that he will soon be well, by allowing his relatives and special friends to cheer him and by having someone to tell him jokes, and let him be solaced also by music on the viol or psaltery. The surgeon must forbid anger, hatred, and sadness in the patient, and remind him that the body grows fat from joy and thin from sadness. He must insist on the patient obeying him faithfully in all things." He repeats with approval the expression of Avicenna that "often the confidence of the patient in his physician does more for the cure of his disease than the physician with all his remedies." Obstinate and conceited patients prone to object to nearly everything that the surgeon wants to do, and who often seem to think that they surpass Galen and Hippocrates in science and wisdom, are likely to delay their cure very much, and they represent the cases with which the surgeon has much difficulty.

Mondeville thought that nursing was extremely important and that without it surgery often failed of its purpose. He says, "For if the assistants are not solicitous and faithful, and obedient to the surgeons in each and every thing which may make for the cure of the disease, they put obstacles and difficulties in the way of the surgeon." It is especially important that the patient's nutrition should be cared for and that the bandages should be managed exactly as the surgeon directs. He has no use for garrulous, talkative nurses, and does not hesitate to say that sometimes near relatives are particularly likely to disturb patients. "Especially are they prone to let drop some hint of bad news which the surgeon may have revealed to them in secret, or even the reports that they may hear from others, friends or enemies, and this provokes the patient to anger or anxiety and is likely to give him fever. If the assistants quarrel among themselves, or are heard murmuring, or if they draw long faces, all of these things will disturb the patients and produce worry and anxiety or fear. The surgeon therefore must be careful in the selection of his nurses, for some of them obey very well while he is present, but do as they like and often just exactly the opposite of what he has directed when he is away."

We do not know enough of the details of Mondeville's life to be sure whether he was married or not.It is probable that he was not, for all of these surgeons of the thirteenth century before Mondeville's time, Theodoric, William of Salicet, Lanfranc, and Guy de Chauliac, after him belonged to the clerical order; Theodoric was a bishop; the others, however, seem only to have been in minor orders. It is therefore from the standpoint of a man who views married life from without that Mondeville makes his remarks as to the difficulty often encountered when wives nurse their husbands. He says that the surgeon has difficulty oftener when husbands or wives care for their spouses than at other times. This is much more likely to take place when the wives are caring for the husbands. "In our days," he says, "in this Gallican part of the world, wives rule their husbands, and the men for the most part permit themselves to be ruled. Whatever a surgeon may order for the cure of a husband then will often seem to the wives to be a waste of good material, though the men seem to be quite willing to get anything that may be ordered for the cure of their wives. The whole cause of this seems to be that every woman seems to think that her husband is not as good as those of other women whom she sees around her." It would be interesting to know how Mondeville was brought to a conclusion so different from modern experience in the matter.

For those who are particularly interested in medical history one of the sections of Henry's book has a special appeal, because he gives in it a sketch of the history of surgery. We are little likely to think, as a rule, that at this time, full two centuries before the close of the Middle Ages, men were interested enough in the doings of those who had gone before them to try to trace the history of the development of their specialty. It is characteristic of the way that the scholarly Mondeville views his own life work that he should have wanted to know something about his predecessors and teach others with regard to them. He begins with Galen, and as Galen divides the famous physicians of the world into three sects, the Methodists, the Empirics, and the Rationalists, so Mondeville divides modern surgery into three sects: first, that of the Salernitans, with Roger, Roland, and the Four Masters;

second, that of William of Salicet and Lanfranc; and third, that of Hugo de Lucca and his brother Theodoric and their modern disciples. He states briefly the characteristics of these three sects. The first limited patients' diet, used no stimulants, dilated all wounds, and got union only after pus formation. The second allowed a liberal diet to weak patients, though not to the strong, but generally interfered with wounds too much. The third believed in a liberal diet, never dilated wounds, never inserted tents, and its members were extremely careful not to complicate wounds of the head by unwise interference. His critical discussion of the three schools is extremely interesting.

Another phase of Mondeville's work that is sympathetic to the moderns is his discussion of the irregular practice of medicine and surgery as it existed in his time. Most of our modern medicine and surgery was anticipated in the olden time; but it may be said that all of the modes of the quack are as old as humanity. Galen's description of the travelling charlatan who settled down in his front yard, not knowing that it belonged to a physician, shows this very well. There were evidently as many of them and as many different kinds in Mondeville's time as in our own. In discussing the opposition that had arisen between physicians and surgeons in his time and their failure to realize that they were both members of a great profession, he enumerates the many different kinds of opponents that the medical profession had. There were "barbers, soothsayers, loan agents, falsifiers, alchemists, meretrices, midwives, old women, converted Jews, Saracens, and indeed most of those who, having wasted their substance foolishly, now proceed to make physicians or surgeons of themselves in order to make their living under the cloak of healing."

What surprises Mondeville however, as it has always surprised every physician who knows the situation, is that so many educated, or at least supposedly well-informed people of the better classes, indeed even of the so-called best classes, allow themselves to be influenced by these quacks. And it is even more surprising to him that so many well-to-do, intelligent people should, for no reason, though without knowledge, presume to give advice in medical matters and especially in even dangerous surgical diseases, and in such delicate affections as diseases of the eyes. "It thus often happens that diseases in themselves curable grow to be simply incurable or are made much worse than they were before." He says that some of the clergymen of his time seemed to think that a knowledge of medicine is infused into them with the sacrament of Holy Orders. He was himself probably a clergyman, and I have in the modern time more than once known of teachers in the clerical seminaries emphasizing this same idea for the clerical students. It is very evident that the world has not changed very much, and that to know any time reasonably well is to find in it comments on the morning paper. We are in the midst of just such a series of interferences with medicine on the part of the clergy as this wise, common-sense surgeon of the thirteenth century deprecated.

In every way Mondeville had the instincts of a teacher. He took advantage of every aid. He was probably the first to use illustrations in teaching anatomy. Guy de Chauliac, whose teacher in anatomy for some time Mondeville was, says in the first chapter of his "Chirurgia Magna" that pictures do not suffice for the teaching of anatomy and that actual dissection is necessary. The passage runs as follows: "In the bodies of men, of apes, and of pigs, and of many other animals, tissues should be studied by dissections and not by pictures, as did Henricus, who was seen to demonstrate anatomy with thirteen pictures."[21] What Chauliac blames is the attempt to replace dissections by pictorial demonstrations. Hyrtl, however, suggests that this invention of Mondeville's was probably very helpful, and was brought about by the impossibility of preserving bodies for long periods as well as the difficulty of obtaining them.

YPERMAN

One of the maxims of the old Greek philosophers was that good is diffusive of itself. As the scholastics put it, *bonum est diffusivum sui.* This proved to be eminently true of the old universities also, and especially of their training in medicine and in surgery. We have the accounts of men from many nations who went to the universities and returned to benefit their own people. Early in the thirteenth century Richard the Englishman was in Italy, having previously been in Paris and probably at Montpellier. Bernard Gordon, probably also an Englishman, was one of the great lights in medicine down at Montpellier, and his book, "Lilium De Medicina," is well known. Two distinguished surgeons whose names have come down to us, having studied in Paris after Lanfranc had created the tradition of great surgical teaching there, came to their homes to be centres of beneficent influence among their people in this matter. One was Yperman, of the town of Ypres in Belgium; the other Ardern of England. Yperman was sent by his fellow-townsmen to Paris in order to study surgery, because they wanted to have a good surgeon in their town and Paris seemed the best school at that time. Ypres was at this period one of the greatest commercial cities of Europe, and probably had a couple of hundred thousand inhabitants. The great hall of the cloth gild, which has been such an attraction for visitors ever since, was built shortly before the town determined upon the very sensible procedure of securing good surgery beyond all doubt by having a townsman specially educated for that purpose.

Yperman's work was practically unknown to us until Broeck, the Belgian historian, discovered manuscript copies of his book on surgery and gathered some details of his life. After his return from Paris, Yperman obtained great renown, which maintained itself in the custom extant in that part of the country even yet of calling an expert surgeon an Yperman. He is the author of two works in Flemish. One of these is a smaller compendium of internal medicine, which is very interesting, however, because it shows the many subjects that were occupying physicians' minds at that time. He treats of dropsy, rheumatism, under which occur the terms coryza and catarrh (the flowing diseases), icterus, phthisis (he calls the tuberculosis, tysiken), apoplexy, epilepsy, frenzy, lethargy, fallen palate, cough, shortness of breath, lung abscess, hemorrhage, blood-spitting, liver abscess, hardening of the spleen, affections of the kidney, bloody urine, diabetes, incontinence of urine, dysuria, strangury, gonorrhea, and involuntary seminal emissions—all these terms are quoted directly from Pagel's account of his work; the original is not available in this country.

JOHN ARDERN

In English-speaking countries of course we are interested in what was done by Englishmen at this time. Fortunately we have the record of one great English surgeon of the period worthy to be placed beside even the writers already mentioned. This is John Ardern, whose name is probably a modification of the more familiar Arden, whose career well deserves attention. I have given a sketch of his work in "The Popes and Science."[22] He was educated at Montpellier, and practised surgery for a time in France. About the middle of the century however, according to Pagel, he went back to his native land and settled for some twenty years at Newark, in Nottinghamshire, and then for nearly thirty years longer, until about the end of the century, was in London. He is the chief representative of English surgery during the Middle Ages. His "Practica," as yet unprinted, contains, according to Pagel, a short sketch of internal medicine, but is mainly devoted to surgery. Contrary to the usual impression with regard to works in medicine and surgery at this time, the book abounds in references to case histories which Ardern had gathered, partly from his own and partly from others' experience. The therapeutic measures that he suggests are usually very simple, in the majority of cases quite rational, though, of course, there are many superstitions among them; but Ardern always furnished a number of suggestions from which to choose. He must have been an expert operator, and had excellent success in the treatment of diseases of the rectum. He seems to have been the first operator who made careful statistics of his cases, and was quite as proud as any modern surgeon of the large numbers that he had operated on, which he gives very exactly. He was the inventor of a new clyster apparatus.

Fortunately we possess here in America, in the Surgeon General's Library at Washington, a very interesting manuscript containing Ardern's surgical writings, though it has not yet been published. Even a little study of this and of the notes on it prepared by an English bibliophile before its purchase by the Surgeon General's Library, serves to show how valuable the work is in the history of surgery. There are illustrations scarcely less interesting than the text. Some of these illustrations were inserted by the original writer or copyist, and some of them later. In general, however, they show a rather high development of the mechanics of surgery at that time. Some of the pages have spaces for illustrations left unfilled, so that evidently the copyist did not complete his work. The titles of certain of the chapters are interesting, as illustrating the fact that our medical and surgical problems were stated clearly in the olden time, and thinking physicians, even six centuries ago, met them quite rationally. There is, for instance, a chapter headed "Against Colic and the Iliac Passion," immediately followed by the subheading, "Method of Administering Clysters." The iliac passion, *passio iliaca* of the old Latin, is usually taken to signify some obstruction of the intestines causing severe pain, vomiting, and eventually fecal vomiting. A good many different forms of severe painful conditions, especially all those complicated by peritonitis, were included under the term, and the modern student of surgery is likely to wonder whether these old observers had not noted that the right iliac region was particularly prone to be the source of fatal conditions. There is a chapter entitled "Against Pain in the Loins and the Kidneys," followed by the chapter subheading, "Against Stone in the Kidneys." There is a chapter with the title, "Against Ulceration of the Bladder or the Kidneys." Another one, with the title "Against Burning of the Urine and Excoriation of the Lower Part of the Yard." Gonorrhea is frankly treated under the name *Shawdepisse,* evidently an English alliteration of the corresponding French word. As to the instrumentation of such conditions and for probing in general, Ardern suggests the use of a lead probe, because it may readily be made to bend any way and not injure the tissues.

MEDIEVAL SURGERY

Even this brief account of the surgeons who taught and studied at the medieval universities demonstrates what fine work they did. It is surely not too much to say that the chapter on university education mainly concerned with them is one of the most interesting in the whole history of the universities. Their story alone is quite enough to refute most of the prevalent impressions and patronizing expressions with regard to medieval education. Their careers serve to show how interested were the men of many nations in the development of an extremely important application of science for the benefit of suffering humanity. Their work utterly contradicts the idea so frequently emphasized that the great students of the Middle Ages were lacking in practicalness. Besides, they make very clear that we have been prone to judge the Middle Ages too much from its speculative philosophies. It has been the custom to say that speculation ruled men's minds and prevented them from making observations, developing science, or applying scientific principles. There was much speculation during the Middle Ages, but probably not any more in proportion than exists at the present day. We were either not acquainted with, or failed to appreciate properly, until comparatively recent years, the other side of medieval accomplishment. Our ignorance led us into misunderstanding of what these generations really did. It was our own fault, because during the Renaissance practically all of these books were edited and printed under the direction of the great scholars of the time in fine editions, but during the eighteenth century nearly all interest was lost in them, and we are only now beginning to get back a certain amount of the precious knowledge that they had in the Renaissance period of this other side of medieval life. We have learned so much about surgery because distinguished scholars devoted themselves to this phase of the history of science. Doubtless there are many other phases of the history of science which suffered the same fate of neglect and with regard to which the future will bring us equally startling revelations. For this reason this marvellous chapter in the history of surgery is a warning as well as a startling record of a marvellous epoch of human progress.

XI

GUY DE CHAULIAC

One of the most interesting characters in the history of medieval medicine, and undoubtedly the most important and significant of these Old-Time Makers of Medicine, is Guy de Chauliac. Most of the false notions so commonly accepted with regard to the Middle Ages at once disappear after a careful study of his career. The idea of the careful application of scientific principles in a great practical way is far removed from the ordinary notion of medieval procedure. Some observations we may concede that they did make, but we are inclined to think that these were not regularly ordered and the lessons of them not drawn so as to make them valuable as experiences. Great art men may have had, but science and, above all, applied science, is a later development of humanity. Particularly is this supposed to be true with regard to the science and practice of surgery, which is assumed to be of comparatively recent origin. Nothing could well be less true, and if the thoroughly practical development of surgery may be taken as a symbol of how capable men were of applying science and scientific principles, then it is comparatively easy to show that the men of the later Middle Ages were occupied very much as have been our recent generations with science and its practical applications.

The immediate evidence of the value of old-time surgery is to be found in the fact that Guy de Chauliac, who is commonly spoken of in the history of medicine as the Father of Modern Surgery, lived his seventy-odd years of life during the fourteenth century and accomplished the best of his work, therefore, some five centuries before surgery in our modern sense of the term is supposed to have developed. A glance at his career, however, will show how old are most of the important developments of surgery, as also in what a thoroughly scientific temper of mind this subject was approached more than a century before the close of the Middle Ages. The life of this French surgeon, indeed, who was a cleric and occupied the position of chamberlain and physician-in-ordinary to three of the Avignon Popes, is not only a contradiction of many of the traditions as to the backwardness of our medieval forbears in medicine, that are readily accepted by many presumably educated people, but it is the best possible antidote for that insistent misunderstanding of the Middle Ages which attributes profound ignorance of science, almost complete failure of observation, and an absolute lack of initiative in applications of science to the men of those times.

Guy de Chauliac's life is modern in nearly every phase. He was educated in a little town of the south of France, made his medical studies at Montpellier, and then went on a journey of hundreds of miles into Italy, in order to make his post-graduate studies. Italy occupied the place in science at that time that Germany has taken during the nineteenth century. A young man who wanted to get into touch with the great masters in medicine naturally went down into the Peninsula. Traditions as to the attitude of the Church to science notwithstanding, Italy where education was more completely under the influence of the Popes and ecclesiastics than in any other country in

Europe, continued to be the home of post-graduate work in science for the next four centuries. Almost needless to say, the journey to Italy was more difficult of accomplishment and involved more expense and time than would even the voyage from America to Europe in our time. Chauliac realized, however, that both time and expense would be well rewarded, and his ardor for the rounding out of his education was amply recompensed by the event. Nor have we any reason for thinking that what he did was very rare, much less unique, in his time. Many a student from France, Germany, and England made the long journey to Italy for post-graduate opportunities during the later Middle Ages.

Even this post-graduate experience in Italy did not satisfy Chauliac, however, for, after having studied several years with the most distinguished Italian teachers of anatomy and surgery, he spent some time in Paris, apparently so as to be sure that he would be acquainted with the best that was being done in his specialty in every part of the world. He then settled down to his own life work, carrying his Italian and French masters' teachings well beyond the point where he received them, and after years of personal experience he gathered together his masters' ideas, tested by his own observations, into his "Chirurgia Magna," a great text-book of surgery which sums up the whole subject succinctly, yet completely, for succeeding generations. When we talk about what he accomplished for surgery, we are not dependent on traditions nor vague information gleaned from contemporaries and successors, who might perhaps have been so much impressed by his personality as to be made over-enthusiastic in their critical judgment of him. We know the man in his surgical works, and they have continued to be classics in surgery ever since. It is an honorable distinction for the medicine of the later fourteenth, the fifteenth, and sixteenth centuries that Guy de Chauliac's book was the most read volume of the time in medicine. Evidently the career of such a man is of import, not alone to physicians, but to all who are interested in the history of education.

Chauliac derives his name from the little town of Chauliac in the diocese of Mende, almost in the centre of what is now the department of Lozère. The records of births and deaths were not considered so important in the fourteenth century as they are now, and so we are not sure of either in the case of Chauliac. It is usually considered that he was born some time during the last decade of the thirteenth century, probably toward the end of it, and that he died about 1370. Of his early education we know nothing, but it must have been reasonably efficient, since it gave him a good working knowledge of Latin, which was the universal language of science and especially of medicine at that time; and though his own style, as must be expected, is no better than that of his contemporaries, he knew how to express his thoughts clearly in straightforward Latin, with only such a mixture of foreign terms as his studies suggested and the exigencies of a new development of science almost required. Later in life he seems to have known Arabic very well, for he is evidently familiar with Arabian books and does not depend merely on translations of them.

Pagel, in the first volume of Puschmann's "Handbook of the History of Medicine," says, on the authority of Nicaise and others, that Chauliac received his early education from the village clergyman. His parents were poor, and but for ecclesiastical interest in him it would have been difficult for him to obtain his education. The Church supplied at that time to a great extent for the foundations and scholarships, home and travelling, of our day, and Chauliac was amongst the favored ones. How well he deserved the favor his subsequent career shows, as it completely justifies the judgment of his patrons. He went first to Toulouse, as we know from his affectionate mention of one of his teachers there. Toulouse was more famous for law, however, than for medicine, and after a time Chauliac sought Montpellier to complete his medical studies.

For English-speaking people an added interest in Guy de Chauliac will be the fact that one of his teachers at Montpellier was Bernard Gordon, very probably a Scotchman, who taught for some thirty-five years at this famous university in the south of France, and died near the end of the first quarter of the fourteenth century. One of Chauliac's fellow-students at Montpellier was John of

Gaddesden, the first English Royal Physician by official appointment of whom we have any account. John is mentioned by Chaucer in his "Doctor of Physic," and is usually looked upon as one of the fathers of English medicine. Chauliac did not think much of him, though his reason for his dislike of him will probably be somewhat startling to those who assume that the men of the Middle Ages always clung servilely to authority. Chauliac's objection to Gaddesden's book is that he merely repeats his masters and does not dare to think for himself. It is not hard to understand that such an independent thinker as Chauliac should have been utterly dissatisfied with a book that did not go beyond the forefathers in medicine that the author quotes. This is the explanation of his well-known expression, "Last of all arose the scentless rose of England ['Rosa Angliæ' was the name of John of Gaddesden's book], in which, on its being sent to me, I hoped to find the odor of sweet originality, but instead of that I encountered only the fictions of Hispanus, of Gilbert, and of Theodoric."

The presence of a Scotch professor and an English fellow-student, afterwards a royal physician, at Montpellier, at the beginning of the fourteenth century, shows how much more cosmopolitan was university life in those times than we are prone to think, and what attraction a great university medical school possessed even for men from long distances.

After receiving his degree of Doctor of Medicine at Montpellier Chauliac went, as we have said, to Bologna. Here he attracted the attention and received the special instruction of Bertruccio, who was attracting students from all over Europe at this time and was making some excellent demonstrations in anatomy, employing human dissections very freely. Chauliac tells of the methods that Bertruccio used in order that bodies might be in as good condition as possible for demonstration purposes, and mentions the fact that he saw him do many dissections in different ways.

In Roth's life of Vesalius, which is usually considered one of our most authoritative medical historical works not only with regard to the details of Vesalius' life, but also in all that concerns anatomy about that time and for some centuries before, there is a passage quoted from Chauliac himself which shows how freely dissection was practised at the Italian universities in the fourteenth century. This passage deserves to be quoted at some length because there are even serious historians who still cite a Bull of Pope Boniface VIII, issued in 1300, forbidding the boiling and dismembering of bodies in order to transport them to long distances for burial in their own country, as being, either rightly or wrongly, interpreted as a prohibition of dissection and, therefore, preventing the development of anatomy. In the notes to his history of dissection during this period in Bologna Roth says: "Without doubt the passage in Guy de Chauliac which tells of having frequently seen dissections, must be considered as referring to Bologna. This passage runs as follows: 'My master Bertruccius conducted the dissection very often after the following manner: the dead body having been placed upon a bench, he used to make four lessons on it. In the first the nutritional portions were treated, because they are so likely to become putrefied. In the second, he demonstrated the spiritual members; in the third, the animate members; in the fourth, the extremities.'" (Roth, "Andreas Vesalius." Basel, 1896.)

Bertruccio's master, Mondino, is hailed in the history of medicine as the father of dissection. His book on dissection was for the next three centuries in the hands of nearly every medical scholar in Europe who was trying to do good work in anatomy. It was not displaced until Vesalius came, the father of modern anatomy, who revolutionized the science in the Renaissance time. Mondino had devoted himself to the subject with unfailing ardor and enthusiasm, and from everywhere in Europe the students came to receive inspiration in his dissecting-room. Within a few years such was the enthusiasm for dissection aroused by him in Bologna that there were many legal prosecutions for body-snatching, the consequence doubtless of a regulation of the Medical Department of the University of Bologna, that if the students brought a body to any of their teachers he was bound to dissect it for them. Bertruccio, Mondino's disciple and successor, continued this great work, and now Chauliac, the third in the tradition, was to carry the Bolognese methods back to France, and his position as chamberlain to the Pope was to give them a wide vogue throughout the world. The great French surgeon's attitude toward anatomy and dissection can be judged from his famous expression that "the surgeon ignorant of anatomy carves the human body as a blind man carves wood." The whole subject of dissection at this time has been fully discussed in the first three chapters of my "Popes and Science," where those who are interested in the matter may follow it to their satisfaction[23].

After his Bologna experience Chauliac went to Paris. Evidently his indefatigable desire to know all that there was to be known would not be satisfied until he had spent some time at the great French university where Lanfranc, after having studied under William of Salicet in Italy, had gone to establish that tradition of French surgery which, carried on so well by Mondeville his great successor, was to maintain Frenchmen as the leading surgeons of the world until the nineteenth century (Pagel). Lanfranc, himself an Italian, had been exiled from his native country, apparently because of political troubles, but was welcomed at Paris because the faculty realized that they needed the inspiration of the Italian medical movement in surgery for the establishment of a good school of surgery in connection with the university. The teaching so well begun by Lanfranc was magnificently continued by Mondeville and Arnold of Villanova and their disciples.

Chauliac was fortunate enough to come under the influence of Petrus de Argentaria, who was worthily maintaining the tradition of practical teaching in anatomy and surgery so well founded by his great predecessors of the thirteenth century. After this grand tour Chauliac was himself prepared to do work of the highest order, for he had been in touch with all that was best in the medicine and surgery of his time.

Like many another distinguished member of his profession, Chauliac did not settle down in the scene of his ultimate labors at once, but was something of a wanderer. His own words are, "*Et per multa tempora operatus fui in multis partibus.*" Perhaps out of gratitude to the clerical patrons of his native town to whom he owed so much, or because of the obligations he considered that he owed them for his education, he practised first in his native diocese of Mende; thence he removed to Lyons, where we know that he lived for several years, for in 1344 he took part as a canon in a chapter that met in the Church of St. Just in that city. Just when he was called to Avignon we do not know, though when the black death ravaged that city in 1348 he was the body-physician of Pope Clement VI, for he is spoken of in a Papal document as "*venerabilis et circumspectus vir, dominus Guido de Cauliaco, canonicus et præpositus ecclesiæ Sancti Justi Lugduni, medicusque domini Nostri Papæ.*" All the rest of his life was passed in the Papal capital, which Avignon was for some seventy years of the fourteenth century. He served as chamberlain-physician to three Popes, Clement VI, Innocent VI, and Urban V. We do not know the exact date of his death, but when Pope Urban V went to Rome in 1367, Chauliac was putting the finishing touches on his "Chirurgia Magna," which, as he tells us, was undertaken as a *solatium senectutis*—a solace in old age. When Urban returned to Avignon for a time in 1370 Chauliac was dead. His life work is summed up for us in this great treatise on surgery, full of anticipations in surgical procedures that we are prone to think much more modern.

Nicaise has emphasized the principles which guided Guy de Chauliac in the choice and interpretation of his authorities by a quotation from Guy himself, which is so different in its tone from what is usually supposed to have been the attitude of mind of the men of science of the time that it would be well for all those who want to understand the Middle Ages better to have it near them. Speaking of the surgeons of his own and immediately preceding generations, Guy says: "One thing particularly is a source of annoyance to me in what these surgeons have written, and it is that they follow one another like so many cranes. For one always says what the other says. I do not know whether it is from fear or from love that they do not deign to listen except to such things as they are accustomed to and as have been proved by authorities. They have to my mind understood very badly Aristotle's second book of metaphysics where he shows that these two things, fear and love, are the greatest obstacles on the road to the knowledge of the truth. Let them give up such friendships and fears. 'Because while Socrates or Plato may be a friend, truth is a greater friend.' Truth is a holy thing and worthy to be honored above everything else. Let them follow the doctrine of Galen, which is entirely made up of experience and reason, and in which one investigates things and despises words."

After all, this is what great authorities in medicine have always insisted on. Once every hundred years or so one finds a really great observer who makes new observations and wakes the world up. He is surprised that men should not have used their powers of observation for themselves, but should have been following old-time masters. His contemporaries often refuse to listen to him at first. His observations, however, eventually make their way. We blame the Middle Ages for following authority, but what have we been always doing but following authority, except for the geniuses who come and lift us out of the rut and illuminate a new portion of the realm of medicine. After they have come, however, and done their work, their disciples proceed to see with their eyes and to think that they are making observations for themselves when they are merely following authority. When the next master in medicine comes along his discovery is neglected because men have not found it in the old books, and usually he has to suffer for daring to have opinions of his own. The fact of the matter is that at any time there is only a very limited number of men who think for themselves. The rest think other people's thoughts and think they are thinking and doing things. As for observation, John Ruskin once said, "Nothing is harder than to see something and tell it simply as you saw it." This is as true in science as in art, and only genius succeeds in doing it well.

Chauliac's book is confessedly a compilation. He has taken the good wherever he found it, though he adds, modestly enough, that his work also contains whatever his own measure of intelligence enabled him to find useful (*quæ juxta modicitatem mei ingenii utilia reputavi*). Indeed it is the critical judgment displayed by Chauliac in selecting from his predecessors that best illustrates at once the practical character of his intellect and his discerning spirit. What the men of his time are said to have lacked is the critical faculty. They were encyclopedic in intellect and gathered all kinds of information without discrimination, is a very common criticism of medieval writers. No one can say this of Chauliac, however, and, above all, he was no respecter of authority, merely for the sake of authority. His criticism of John of Gaddesden's book shows that the blind following of those who had gone before was his special *bête noir*. His bitterest reproach for many of his predecessors was that "they follow one another like cranes, whether for love or fear, I cannot say."

Chauliac's right to the title of father of surgery will perhaps be best appreciated from the brief account of his recommendations as to the value of surgical intervention for conditions in the three most important cavities of the body, the skull, the thorax, and the abdomen. These cavities have usually been the dread of surgeons. Chauliac not only used the trephine, but laid down very exact indications for its application. Expectant treatment was to be the rule in wounds of the head, yet when necessary, interference was counselled as of great value. His prognosis of brain injuries was much better than that of his predecessors. He says that he had seen injuries of the brain followed by some loss of brain substance, yet with complete recovery of the patient. In one case that he notes a considerable amount of brain substance was lost, yet the patient recovered with only a slight defect of memory, and even this disappeared after a time. He lays down exact indications for the opening of the thorax, that *noli me tangere* of surgeons at all times, even our own, and points out the relations of the ribs and the diaphragm, so as to show just where the opening should be made in order to remove fluid of any kind.

In abdominal conditions, however, Chauliac's anticipation of modern views is most surprising. He recognized that wounds of the intestines were surely fatal unless leakage could be prevented. Accordingly he suggested the opening of the abdomen and the sewing up of such intestinal wounds as could be located. He describes a method of suture for these cases and seems, like many another abdominal surgeon, even to have invented a special needleholder.

To most people it would seem absolutely out of the question that such surgical procedures could be practised in the fourteenth century. We have the definite record of them, however, in a text-book that was the most read volume on the subject for several centuries. Most of the surprise with regard to these operations will vanish when it is recalled that in Italy during the thirteenth century, as we have already seen, methods of anæsthesia by means of opium and mandragora were in common use, having been invented in the twelfth century and perfected by Ugo da Lucca, and Chauliac must not only have known but must have frequently employed various methods of anæsthesia.

In discussing amputations he has described in general certain methods of anæsthesia in use in his time, and especially the method by means of inhalaion. It would not seem to us in the modern time that this method would be very successful, but there is an enthusiastic accord of authorities attesting that operations were done at this time with the help of this inhalant without the infliction of pain. Chauliac says:

> "Some prescribe medicaments which send the patient to sleep, so that the incision may not be felt, such as opium, the juice of the morel, hyoscyamus, mandrake, ivy, hemlock, lettuce. A new sponge is soaked by them in these juices and left to dry in the sun; and when they have need of it they put this sponge into warm water and then hold it under the nostrils of the patient until he goes to sleep. Then they perform the operation."

Many people might be prone to think that the hospitals of Chauliac's time would not be suitable for such surgical work as he describes. It is, however, only another amusing assumption of this self-complacent age of ours to think that we were the first who ever made hospitals worthy of the name and of the great humanitarian purpose they subserve. As a matter of fact, the old-time hospitals were even better than ours or, as a rule, better than any we had until the present generation. In "The Popes and Science," in the chapter on "The Foundation of City Hospitals," I call attention to the fact that architects of the present day go back to the hospitals of the Middle Ages in order to find the models for hospitals for the modern times. Mr. Arthur Dillon, a well-known New York architect, writing of a hospital built at Tonnerre in France, toward the end of the thirteenth century (1292), says:

"It was an admirable hospital in every way, and it is doubtful if we to-day surpass it. It was isolated; the ward was separated from the other buildings; it had the advantage we so often lose of being but one story high, and more space was given to each patient than we can now afford.

"The ventilation by the great windows and ventilators in the ceiling was excellent; it was cheerfully lighted; and the arrangement of the gallery shielded the patients from dazzling light and from draughts from the windows and afforded an easy means of supervision, while the division by the roofless low partitions isolated the sick and obviated the depression that comes from sight of others in pain.

"It was, moreover, in great contrast to the cheerless white wards of to-day. The vaulted ceiling was very beautiful;

the woodwork was richly carved, and the great windows over the altars were filled with colored glass. Altogether it was one of the best examples of the best period of Gothic Architecture."[24]

The fine hospital thus described was but one of many. Virchow, in his article on hospitals quoted in the same chapter, called attention to the fact that in the thirteenth and fourteenth centuries every town of five thousand or more inhabitants had its hospital, founded on the model of the great Santo Spirito Hospital in Rome, and all of them did good work. The surgeons of Guy de Chauliac's time would indeed find hospitals wherever they might be called in consultation, even in small towns. They were more numerous in proportion to population than our own and, as a rule, at least as well organized as ours were until the last few years.

It is no wonder that with such a good hospital organization excellent surgery was accomplished. Hernia was Chauliac's specialty, and in it his surgical judgment is admirable. Mondeville before his time did not hesitate to say that many operations for hernia were done not for the benefit of the patient, but for the benefit of the surgeon,—a very striking anticipation of remarks that one sometimes hears even at the present time. Chauliac discussed operations for hernia very conservatively. His rule was that a truss should be worn, and no operation attempted unless the patient's life was endangered by the hernia. It is to him that we owe the invention of a well-developed method of taxis, or manipulation of a hernia, to bring about its reduction, which was in use until the end of the nineteenth century. He suggested that trusses could not be made according to rule, but must be adapted to each individual case. He invented several forms of truss himself, and in general it may be said that his manipulative skill and his power to apply his mechanical principles to his work are the most characteristic of his qualities. This is particularly noteworthy in his chapters on fractures and dislocations, in which he suggests various methods of reduction and realizes very practically the mechanical difficulties that were to be encountered in the correction of the deformities due to these pathological conditions. In a word, we have a picture of the skilled surgeon of the modern time in this treatise of a fourteenth-century teacher of surgery.

Chauliac discusses six different operations for the radical cure of hernia. As Gurlt points out, he criticises them from the same standpoint as that of recent surgeons. The object of radical operations for hernia is to produce a strong, firm tissue support over the ring through which the cord passes, so that the intestines cannot descend through it. It is rather interesting to find that the surgeons of this time tried to obliterate the canal by means of the cautery, or inflammation producing agents, arsenic and the like, a practice that recalls some methods still used more or less irregularly. They also used gold wire, which was to be left in the tissues and is supposed to protect and strengthen the closure of the ring. At this time all these operations for the radical cure of hernia involved the sacrifice of the testicle because the old surgeons wanted to obliterate the ring completely, and thought this the easiest way. Chauliac discusses the operation in this respect and says that he has seen many cases in which men possessed of but one testicle have procreated, and this is a case where the lesser of two evils is to be chosen.

Of course Guy de Chauliac would not have been able to operate so freely on hernia and suggest, following his own experience, methods of treatment of penetrating wounds of the abdomen only that he had learned the lessons of antiseptic surgery which had been gradually developed among the great surgeons of Italy during the preceding century. The use of the stronger wines as a dressing together with insistence on the most absolute cleanliness of the surgeon before the operation, and careful details of cleanliness during the operation, made possible the performance of many methods of surgical intervention that would otherwise surely have been fatal. Probably nothing is harder to understand than that after these practical discoveries men should have lost sight of their significance, and after having carefully studied the viscous exudation which produces healthy natural union, should have come to the thought of the necessity for the formation of laudable pus before union might be expected. The mystery is really no greater than that of many another similar incident in human history, but it strikes us more forcibly because the discovery and gradual development of antiseptic surgery in our own time has meant so much for us. Already even in Chauliac's practice, however, some of the finer elements of the technique that made surgery antiseptic to a marked degree, if not positively aseptic in many cases, were not being emphasized as they were by his predecessors, and there was a beginning of surgical meddlesomeness reasserting itself.

It must not be thought, however, that it was only with the coarse applications of surgery that Chauliac concerned himself. He was very much interested in the surgical treatment of eye diseases and wrote a monograph on cataract, in which he gathers what was known before his time and discusses it in the light of his own experience. The writing of such a book is not so surprising at this time if we recall that in the preceding century the famous Pope John XXI, who had been a physician before he became Pope, and under the name of Peter of Spain was looked up to as one of the distinguished scientists of his time, had written a book on eye diseases that has recently been the subject of much attention.

Pope John had much to say of cataract, dividing it into traumatic and spontaneous, and suggesting the needling of cataract, a gold needle being used for the purpose. Chauliac's method of treating cataract was by depression. His care in the selection of patients may be appreciated from his treatment of John of Luxembourg, King of Bavaria, blind from cataract, who consulted Chauliac in 1336 while on a visit to Avignon with the King of France.

Chauliac refused to operate, however, and put off the King with dietary regulations.

In the chapter on John of Arcoli and Medieval Dentistry we call attention to the fact that Chauliac discussed dental surgery briefly, yet with such practical detail as to show very clearly how much more was known about this specialty in his time than we have had any idea of until recent years. He recognized the dentists as specialists, calls them dentatores, but thinks that they should operate under the direction of a physician—hence the physician should know much about teeth and especially about their preservation. He enumerates instruments that dentists should have and shows very clearly that the specialty had reached a high state of development. A typical example of Chauliac's common sense and dependence on observation and not tradition is to be found in what he has to say with regard to methods of removing the teeth without the use of extracting instruments. It is characteristic of his method of dealing with traditional remedies, even though of long standing, that he brushes them aside with some impatience if they have not proved themselves in his experience.

> "The ancients mention many medicaments, which draw out the teeth without iron instruments or which make them more easy to draw out; such as the milky juice of the tithymal with pyrethrum, the roots of the mulberry and caper, citrine arsenic, aqua fortis, the fat of forest frogs. But these

> remedies promise much and accomplish but little — mais ils donnent beaucoup de promesses, et peu, d'opérations."

It is no wonder that Chauliac has been enthusiastically praised. Nicaise has devoutly gathered many of these praises into a sheaf of eulogies at the end of his biography of the great French surgeon. He tells us that Fallopius compared him to Hippocrates. John Calvo of Valencia, who translated the "Great Surgery" into Spanish, looks upon him as the first law-giver of surgery. Freind, the great English physician, in 1725 called him the Prince of Surgeons. Ackermann said that Guy de Chauliac's text-book will take the place of all that has been written on the subject down to his time, so that even if all the other works had been lost his would replace them. Dezimeris, commenting on this, says that "if one should take this appreciation literally, this surgeon of the fourteenth century would be the first and, up to the present time, the only author who ever merited such an eulogy." "At least," he adds, "we cannot refuse him the distinction of having made a work infinitely superior to all those which appeared up to this time and even for a long time afterwards. Posterity rendered him this justice, for he was for three centuries the classic *par excellence*. He rendered the study easy and profitable, and all the foreign nations the tributaries of our country." Peyrihle considered Guy's "Surgery" as the most valuable and complete work of all those of the same kind that had been published since Hippocrates and added that the reading of it was still useful in his time in 1784. Bégin, in his work on Ambroise Paré, says "that Guy has written an immortal book to which are attached the destinies of French surgeons."

Malgaigne, in his "History of Surgery," does not hesitate to say, "I do not fear to say that, Hippocrates alone excepted, there is not a single treatise on surgery,—Greek, Latin, or Arabic,—which I place above, or even on the same level with, this magnificent work, 'The Surgery of Guy de Chauliac.'" Daremberg said, "Guy seems to us a surgeon above all erudite, yet expert and without ever being rash. He knows, above all, how to choose what is best in everything." Verneuil, in his "Conférence sur Les Chirurgiens Érudits," says, "The services rendered by the 'Great Surgery' were immense; by it there commenced for France an era of splendor. It is with justice, then, that posterity has decreed to Guy de Chauliac the title of Father of French surgery."

The more one reads of Chauliac's work the less is one surprised at the estimation in which he has been held wherever known. It would not be hard to add a further sheaf of compliments to those collected by Nicaise. Modern writers on the history of medicine have all been enthusiastic in their admiration of him, just in proportion to the thoroughness of their acquaintance with him. Portal, in his "History of Anatomy and Surgery," says, "Finally, it may be averred that Guy de Chauliac said nearly everything which modern surgeons say, and that his work is of infinite price but unfortunately too little read, too little pondered." Malgaigne declares Chauliac's "Chirurgia Magna" to be "a masterpiece of learned and luminous writing." Professor Clifford Allbutt, the Regius Professor of Physic at the University of Cambridge, says of Chauliac's treatise: "This great work I have studied carefully and not without prejudice; yet I cannot wonder that Fallopius compared the author to Hippocrates or that John Freind calls him the Prince of Surgeons. It is rich, aphoristic, orderly, and precise."[25]

If to this account of his professional career it be added that Chauliac's personality is, if possible, more interesting than his surgical accomplishment, some idea of the significance of the life of the great father of modern surgery will be realized. We have already quoted the distinguished words of praise accorded him by Pope Clement VI. That they were well deserved, Chauliac's conduct during the black death which ravaged Avignon in 1348, shortly after his arrival in the Papal City, would have been sufficient of itself to attest. The occurrence of the plague in a city usually gave rise to an exhibition of the most arrant cowardice, and all who could, fled. In many of the European cities the physicians joined the fugitives, and the ailing were left to care for themselves. With a few notable exceptions, this was the case at Avignon, but Guy was among those who remained faithful to his duty and took on himself the self-sacrificing labor of caring for the sick, doubly harassing because so many of his brother physicians were absent. He denounces their conduct as shameful, yet does not boast of his own courage, but on the contrary says that he was in constant fear of the disease. Toward the end of the epidemic he was attacked by the plague and for a time his life was despaired of. Fortunately he recovered, to become the most influential among his colleagues, the most highly admired of the physicians of his generation, and the close personal friend of all the high ecclesiastics, who had witnessed his magnificent display of courage and of helpfulness for the plague-stricken during the epidemic. He wrote a very clear account of the epidemic, which leaves no doubt that it was true bubonic plague.

After this fine example, Chauliac's advice to brother physicians in the specialty of surgery carried added weight. In the Introductory chapter of his "Chirurgia Magna" he said:

> "The surgeon should be learned, skilled, ingenious, and of good morals. Be bold in things that are sure, cautious in dangers; avoid evil cures and practices; be gracious to the sick, obliging to his colleagues, wise in his predictions. Be chaste, sober, pitiful, and merciful; not covetous nor extortionate of money; but let the recompense be moderate, according to the work, the means of the sick, the character of the issue or event, and its dignity."

No wonder that Malgaigne says of him, "Never since Hippocrates has medicine heard such language filled with so much nobility and so full of matter in so few words."

Chauliac was in every way worthy of his great contemporaries and the period in which his lot was cast. Ordinarily we are not apt to think of the early fourteenth century as an especially productive period in human history, but such it is. Dante's Divine Comedy was entirely written during Chauliac's life. Petrarch was born within a few years of Chauliac himself; Boccaccio in Italy, and Chaucer in England, wrote while Chauliac was still alive. Giotto did his great painting, and his pupils were laying the deep, firm foundations of modern art. Many of the great cathedrals were being finished. Most of the universities were in the first flush of their success as moulders of the human mind. There are few centuries in history that can show the existence of so many men whose work was to have an enduring influence for all the after time as this upon which Chauliac's career shed so bright a light. The preceding century had seen the origin of the universities and the rise of such supremely great men as Albertus Magnus, Roger Bacon, Thomas Aquinas, and the other famous scholars of the early days of the mendicant orders, and had made the intellectual mould of university training in which men's minds for seven centuries were to be formed, so that Chauliac, instead of being an unusual phenomenon is only a fitting expression of the interest of this time in everything, including the physical sciences and, above all, medicine and surgery.

For some people it may be a source of surprise that Chauliac should have had the intellectual training to enable him to accomplish such judicious work in his specialty. Many people will be apt to assume that he accomplished what he did in spite of his training, genius succeeding even in an unfavorable environment, and notwithstanding educational disadvantages. Those who would be satisfied with any such explanation, however, know nothing of the educational opportunities provided in the period of which Chauliac was the fruit. He is a typical university man of the beginning of the fourteenth century, and the universities must be given due credit for him. It is ordinarily assumed that the universities paid very little attention to science and that scientists would find practically nothing to satisfy in their curricula. Professor Huxley in his address on "Universities, Actual and Ideal," delivered as the Rectorial Address at Aberdeen University in 1874, declared that they were probably educating in the real sense of the word better than we do now. (See quotation in "The Medical School at Salerno.")

In the light of Chauliac's life it is indeed amusing to read the excursions of certain historians into the relationship of the Popes and the Church to science during the Middle Ages. Chauliac is typically representative of medieval science, a man who gave due weight to authority, yet tried everything by his own experience, and who sums up in himself such wonderful advance in surgery that during the last twenty years the students of the history of medicine have been more interested in him than in anyone who comes during the intervening six centuries. Chauliac, however, instead of meeting with any opposition, encountered encouragement, liberal patronage, generous interest, and even enjoyed the intimate friendship of the highest ecclesiastics and the Popes of his time. In every way his life may be taken as a type of what we have come to know about the Middle Ages, when we know them as we should, in the lives of the men who counted for most in them, and do not accept merely the broad generalizations which are always likely to be deceptive and which in the past have led men into the most absurd and ridiculous notions with regard to a wonderful period in human history.

That Guy de Chauliac was no narrow specialist is abundantly evident from his book, for while the "Great Surgery" treats of the science and art of surgery as its principal subject, there are remarks about nearly everything else relating to medicine, and most of them show a deep interest, a thorough familiarity, and an excellent judgment. Besides we have certain expressions with regard to intellectual matters generally which serve to show Guy as a profound thinker, who thoroughly appreciated just how accumulations of knowledge came to men and how far each generation or member of a generation should go and yet how limited must, after all, be the knowledge obtained by any one person. With regard to books, for instance, he said, "for everyone cannot have all the books, and even if he did have them it would be too tiresome to read them all and completely, and it would require a godlike memory to retain them all." He realized, however, that each generation, provided it took the opportunities offered it, was able to see a little bit farther than its predecessor, and the figure that he employs to express this is rather striking. "Sciences," he said, "are made by additions. It is quite impossible that the man who begins a science should finish it. We are like infants, clinging to the neck of a giant; for we can see all the giant sees and a little more."

One of the most interesting features of the history of Guy de Chauliac is the bibliography of his works which has been written by Nicaise. This is admirably complete, labored over with the devotion that characterized Nicaise's attitude of unstinted admiration for the subject. Altogether he has some sixty pages of a quarto volume with regard to the various editions of Guy's works.

The first manuscript edition of Guy de Chauliac was issued in 1363, the first printed edition in 1478. Even in the fourteenth century Guy's great work was translated into all the languages generally used in Europe. Nicaise succeeded in placing 34 complete manuscripts of the "Great Surgery": 22 of these are in Latin, 4 are in French, 3 are in English, 2 only in Provençal, though that was the language spoken in the region where much of Chauliac's life was passed, and one each in Italian, in Low Dutch, and in Hebrew. Of the English manuscripts, one is number twenty-five English of the Bibliothèque Nationale, Paris; a second is number 3666 English of the Sloane collection in the British Museum, and a third is in the Library of the University of Cambridge.[26]

Paulin Paris, probably one of the best of recent authorities on the age and significance of old manuscripts, says in the third volume of his "Manuscrits Français," page 346, "This manuscript [of Guy de Chauliac's "Great Surgery"] was made, if not during the life, then certainly very shortly after the death of the author. It is one of the oldest that can be cited, and the fact that an English translation was made so near to the time of the original composition of the book attests the great reputation enjoyed by Guy de Chauliac at this time, and which posterity has fully confirmed."

The Sloane copy in the British Museum contains some medical recipes at the end by Francis Verney. It was probably written in the fifteenth century. Its title is:

> "The inventorie or the collectorie in cirurgicale parte of medicine compiled and complete in the yere of our Lord 1363, with some additions of other doctours, necessary to the foresaid arte or crapte (crafte?)."[27]

What we find in the period of manuscripts, however, is as nothing compared to the prestige of Guy de Chauliac's work, once the age of printing began. Nicaise was able to find sixty different printed editions of the "Great Surgery." Nine others that are mentioned by authors have disappeared and apparently no copies of them are in existence. Besides there are sixty editions of portions of the work, of compendiums of it and commentaries on it. Altogether 129 editions are extant. Of these there are sixteen Latin editions, forty-three French, five Italian, four Low Dutch, five Catalan, and one English. Fourteen appeared in the fifteenth century, thirty-eight in the sixteenth century, and seventeen in the seventeenth century. The fourteen editions belonging to the *incunabula* of printing, issued, that is, before the end of the fifteenth century, show what lively interest there was in the French surgeon of the preceding century, since printing presses at this precious time were occupied only with the books that were considered indispensable for scholars. The first edition of the "Great Surgery" was printed in 1478 at Lyons. Printing had only been introduced there five years before. This first edition, *primus primarius* or *editio princeps,* was a French translation by Nicholas Panis. In 1480 an Italian edition was printed at Venice. The first Latin edition was printed also in Venice in 1490.

It would be only natural to expect that the successors of Guy de Chauliac, and especially those who had come personally in contact with him, would take advantage of his thorough work to make still further advances in surgery. As matter of fact, decadence in surgery is noted immediately after his death. Three men taught at the University of Montpellier at the end of the fourteenth and the beginning of the fifteenth century, John de Tornamira, Valesco de Taranta, and John Faucon. They cannot be compared, Gurlt says, with Guy de Chauliac, though they were physicians of reputation in their time. Faucon made a compendium of Guy's work for students. Somehow there seemed to be the impression that surgery had now reached a point of development beyond which it could not advance. Unfortunate political conditions, wars, the withdrawal of the Popes from Avignon to Rome, and other disturbances, distracted men's minds, and surgery deteriorated to a considerable extent, until the new spirit at the time of the Renaissance came to inject fresh life into it.

XII

MEDIEVAL DENTISTRY – GIOVANNI OF ARCOLI

If there is one phase of our present-day medicine and surgery that most of us are likely to be quite sure is of very recent development it is dentistry. Probably most people would declare at once that they had every reason to think that the science and art of dentistry, as we have it now, developed for the first time in the world's history during the last generation or two. It is extremely interesting to realize then, in the light of this almost universal persuasion, founded to a great extent on the conviction that man is in process of evolution and that as a consequence we must surely be doing things now that men never did before, to find that dentistry, both as an art and science, is old; that it has developed at a number of times in the world's history, and that as fortunately for history its work was done mainly in indestructible materials, the teeth themselves and metal prosthetic apparatus, we have actual specimens of what was accomplished at a number of periods in the olden times.

Surprising as it will seem to those who hear of it for the first time, dentistry reached high perfection even in what we know as ancient history. It is rather easy to trace scientific and craftsmanlike interest in it during the medieval period and in the magnificent development of surgery that came just at the end of the Middle Ages, dentistry shared to such degree that some of the text-books of the writers on surgery of this time furnish abundant evidence of anticipations of many of the supposedly most modern developments of dentistry.

There are a number of historical traditions with regard to dentistry and the treatment of the teeth in Egypt that can be traced back to good authorities in Egyptology of a generation or more ago, but it is rather hard to confirm the accounts we have by actual specimens; either none were found or for some reason those actually discovered are now not readily available for study. Among the Phenicians however, though we have good reasons to think that they learned their arts and crafts from the Egyptians, there is convincing evidence of a high development of dentistry. M. Ernest Renan, during an exploring expedition in Phenicia, found in the old necropolis at Sidon a set of teeth wired together, two of which were artificial. It was a striking example of bridgework, very well done, and may now be seen in the Louvre. It would be more than a little surprising, from what we know of the lack of inventiveness on the part of the Phenicians and their tendency to acquire their arts by imitation, if they had reached such a climax of invention by themselves. Since they adapted and adopted most of their arts and crafts from Egypt, with which they were in close commercial relations, it has been argued with some plausibility that the Egyptians may have had many modes of dental prosthesis, but removed all artificial teeth and dental appliances from the mouth of corpses before embalming them, in preparation for the next world, because there was some religious objection to such human handiwork being left in place for the hereafter, as they hoped for it.

There is a well-authenticated tradition of intimate intercourse in a commercial way between the old Etruscans who inhabited the Italian hill country and the Phenicians, so that it is no surprise to find that the oldest of Etruscan tombs contain some fine examples of bridgework. An improvement has come over Phenician work however, and bands of gold instead of wire are used for holding artificial teeth in place. Guerini, whose "History of Dentistry" is the standard work on the subject, on a commission from the Italian government, carefully studied these specimens of Etruscan dental work in the museums of Italy, and has made some interesting observations on them. In one specimen, which is especially notable, two incisor teeth are replaced by a single tooth from a calf. This was grooved in such a way as to make it seem like two separate teeth. Guerini suggests a very interesting and quite unexpected source for this. While examining the specimen he wondered where the old

Etruscan dentist had obtained a calf's tooth without a trace of wear on it. He came to the conclusion that he must have cut into the gums of a young calf before the permanent tooth was erupted in order to get this structure absolutely unworn for his purpose. A number of examples of bridgework have been found in the old Etruscan tombs. The dates of their construction are probably not later than 500 B.C., and some of them are perhaps earlier than 700 B.C.

The Etruscans affected the old Romans in the matter of dentistry, so that it is easy to understand the passage in the "Laws of the Twelve Tables," issued about 450 B.C., which, while forbidding the burial of gold with corpses, made a special exception for such gold as was fastened to the teeth. Gold was rare at Rome, and care was exercised not to allow any unnecessary decrease of the visible supply almost in the same way as governments now protect their gold reserves. It may seem like comparing little things with great, but the underlying principle is the same. Hence this special law and its quite natural exception.

In Pope Julius' Museum in Rome there is a specimen of a gold cap made of two plates of gold riveted together and also riveted to bands of metal which were fastened around the neighboring teeth in order to hold the cap in place. This is from later Republican times at Rome. At the end of the Republic and the beginning of the Empire there appear to have been many forms of dental appliances. Martial says that the reason why one lady's teeth—whose name he does not conceal—are white and another's—name also given—were dark, was that the first one bought hers and the second still had her own. In another satiric poem he describes an elderly woman as so much frightened that when she ran away her teeth fell out, while her friends lost their false hair. Fillings of many kinds were used, dentrifices of nearly every kind were invented, and dentistry evidently reached a high stage of development,though we have nowhere a special name for dentist, and the work seems to have been done by physicians, who took this as a specialty.

While in the Middle Ages there was, owing to conditions, a loss of much of this knowledge of antiquity with regard to dentistry, or an obscuration of it, it never disappeared completely, and whenever men have written seriously about medicine, above all about surgery in relation to the face and the mouth, the teeth have come in for their share of scientific and practical consideration. Aëtius, the first important Christian writer on medicine and surgery, discusses, as we have seen in the sketch of him, the nutrition of the teeth, their nerves, "which came from the third pair and entered the teeth by a small hole existing at the end of the root," and other interesting details of anatomy and physiology. He knows much about the hygiene of the teeth, discusses extraction and the cure of fistula and other details. Paul of Ægina in the next century has much more, and while they both quote mainly from older authors there seems no doubt that they themselves had made not a few observations and had practical experience.

It was from these men that the Arabian physicians and surgeons obtained their traditions of medicine, and so it is not surprising to find that they discuss dental diseases and their treatment rationally and in considerable detail. Abulcasis particularly has much that is of significance and interest. We have pictures of two score of dental instruments that were used by them. The Arabs not only treated and filled carious teeth and even replaced those that were lost, but they also corrected deformities of the mouth and of the dental arches. Orthodontia is sometimes said to be of much later origin and to begin many centuries after Abulcasis' time, yet no one who knows of his work can speak of Orthodontia as an invention after him. In this, however, as in most of the departments of medicine and surgery, the Arabs were merely imitators, though probably they expanded somewhat the practical knowledge that had come to them.

When the great revival in surgery came in the twelfth and thirteenth centuries it is not surprising that there should also have been an important renewal of interest in dentistry. A detailed review of this would take us too far afield, but at least something may be said of two or three of the great representative surgical writers who touched on this specialty.

About the middle of the fourteenth century that prince of surgeons, and model of surgical writers, Guy de Chauliac, wrote his great text-book of surgery, "Le Grande Chirurgie." An extremely interesting feature of this work is to be found in the chapters that treat of diseases of the teeth. These are not very comprehensive, and are evidently not so much the result of his experience, as the fruit of his reading, yet they contain many practical valuable ideas that are supposed to be ever so much later than the middle of the fourteenth century. His anatomy and physiology at least are not without many errors. His rules for the preservation of the teeth show that the ordinary causes of dental decay were well recognized even as early as this. Emphasis was laid on not taking foods too hot or too cold, and above all not to follow either hot or cold food by something very different from it in temperature. The breaking of hard things with the teeth was recognized as one of the most frequent causes of such deterioration of the enamel as gives opportunity for the development of decay. The eating of sweets, and especially the sticky sweets—preserves and the like—was recognized as an important source of caries. The teeth were supposed to be cleaned frequently, and not to be cleaned too roughly, for this would do more harm than good. We find these rules repeated by succeeding writers on general surgery, who touch upon dentistry, or at least the care of the teeth, and they were not original with Guy de Chauliac, but part of the tradition of surgery.

As noted by Guerini in his "History of Dentistry," the translation of which was published under the auspices of the National Dental Association of the United States of America,[28] Chauliac recognized the dentists as specialists. Besides, it should be added, as is evident from his enumeration of the surgical instruments which he declares necessary for them, they were not as we might easily think in the modern time mere tooth pullers, but at least the best among them treated teeth as far as their limited knowledge and means at command enabled them to do so, and these means were much more elaborate than we have been led to think, and much more detailed than we have reason to know that they were at certain subsequent periods.

In fact, though Guy de Chauliac frankly confesses that he touches on the subject of dentistry only in order to complete his presentation of the subject of surgery and not because he has anything of his own to say with regard to the subject, there is much that is of present-day interest in his brief paragraphs. He observes that operations on the teeth are special and belong to the *dentatores,* or dentists, to whom doctors had given them over. He considers, however, that the operations in the mouth should be performed under the direction of a physician. It is in order to give physicians the general principles with which they may be able to judge of the advisability or necessity for dental operations that his short chapters are written. If their advice is to be of value, physicians should know the various methods of treatment suitable for dental diseases, including mouth washes, gargles, masticatories, anointments, rubbings, fumigations, cauterizations, fillings, filings, and the various manual operations. He says that the *dentator* must be provided with the appropriate instruments, among which he names scrapers, rasps, straight and curved spatumina, elevators, simple and with two branches, toothed tenacula, and many different forms of probes and canulas. He should also have small scalpels, tooth trephines, and files.

Chauliac is particularly emphatic in his insistence on not permitting alimentary materials to remain in cavities, and suggests that if cavities between the teeth tend to retain food material they should even be filed in such a way as to prevent these accumulations. His directions for cleansing the teeth were rather detailed. His favorite treatment for wounds was wine, and he knew that he succeeded by means of it in securing union by first intention. It is not surprising, then, to find that he recommends rinsing of the mouth with wine as a precaution against dental decay. A vinous decoction of wild mint and of pepper he considered particularly beneficial, though he thought that dentifrices, either powder or liquid, should also be used. He seems to recommend the powder dentifrices as more efficacious. His favorite prescription for a tooth powder, while more elaborate, resembles to such an extent, at least some, if not indeed most of those, that are used at the present time, that it seems worth while giving his directions for it. He took equal parts of cuttle bone, small white sea-shells, pumice stone, burnt stag's horn, nitre, alum, rock salt, burnt roots of iris, aristolochia, and reeds. All of these substances should be carefully reduced to powder and then mixed. His favorite liquid dentifrice contained the following ingredients,—half a pound each of sal ammoniac and rock salt, and a quarter of a pound of sacharin alum. All these were to be reduced to powder and placed in a glass alembic and dissolved. The teeth should be rubbed with it, using a little scarlet cloth for the purpose. Just why this particular color of cleansing cloth was recommended is not quite clear.

He recognized, however, that cleansing of the teeth properly often became impossible by any scrubbing method, no matter what the dentifrice used, because of the presence of what we call tartar and what he called hardened limosity or limyness (*limosité endurcie*). When that condition is present he suggests the use of rasps and spatumina and other instrumental means of removing the tartar.

Evidently he did not believe in the removal of the teeth unless this was absolutely necessary and no other method of treatment would avail to save the patient from continuous distress. He summarizes the authorities with regard to the extraction of teeth and the removal of dental fragments and roots. He evidently knew of the many methods suggested before his time of removing teeth without recourse to instrumental extraction. There were a number of applications to the gums that were claimed by older authors to remove the teeth without the need of metal instruments. We might expect that Chauliac would detect the fallacy with regard to these and expose it. He says that while much is claimed for these methods he has never seen them work in practice and he distrusts them entirely.

The most interesting phase of what Guy de Chauliac has to say with regard to dentistry is of course to be found in his paragraphs on the artificial replacement of lost teeth and the subject of dental prosthesis generally. When teeth become loose he advises that they be fastened to the healthy ones with a gold chain. Guerini suggests that he evidently means a gold wire. If the teeth fall out they may be replaced by the teeth of another person or with artificial teeth made from oxbone, which may be fixed in place by a fine metal ligature. He says that such teeth may be serviceable for a long while. This is a rather curt way of treating so large a subject as dental prosthesis, but it contains a lot of suggestive material. He was quoting mainly the Arabian authors, and especially Abulcasis and Ali Abbas and Rhazes, and these of course, as we have said, mentioned many methods of artificially replacing teeth as also of transplantation and of treatment of the deformities of the dental arches.

On the whole, however, it must be confessed that we have here in the middle of the fourteenth century a rather surprising anticipation of the knowledge of a special department of medicine which is usually considered to be distinctly modern, and indeed as having only attracted attention seriously in comparatively recent times.

After Guy de Chauliac the next important contributor to dentistry is Giovanni of Arcoli, often better known by his Latin name, Johannes Arculanus, who was a professor of medicine and surgery at Bologna and afterwards at Padua, just before and after the middle of the fifteenth century, and who died in 1484. He is famous principally for being the first we know who mentions the filling of teeth with gold.

It might possibly be suggested that coming at this time Arculanus should rather be reckoned as a Maker of Medicine in the Renaissance than as belonging to the Middle Ages and its influences. His education, however, was entirely completed before the earliest date at which the Renaissance movement is usually said to begin, that is with the fall of Constantinople in 1452, and he was dead before the other date, that of the discovery of America in 1492, which the Germans have in recent years come to set down as the end of the Middle Ages. Besides, what he has to say about dentistry occurs in typical medieval form. It is found in a commentary on Rhazes, written just about the middle of the fifteenth century. In the later true

Renaissance such a commentary would have been on a Greek author. In his commentary Arculanus touches on most of the features of medicine and surgery from the standpoint of his own experience as well as from what he knows of the writings of his predecessors and contemporaries. With the rest he has a series of chapters on diseases of the teeth. Guerini in his "History of Dentistry" says that "this subject [dentistry] is treated rather fully, and with great accuracy." Even some short references to it will, I think, demonstrate this rather readily.[29]

Arculanus is particularly full in his directions for the preservation of the teeth. We are rather prone to think that prophylaxis is comparatively a modern idea, and that most of the principles of conservation of human tissues and the prevention of deterioration and disease are distinctly modern. It needs only a little consideration of Arculanus' instruction in the matter of the teeth, however, to undo any such false impression. For obvious reasons I prefer to quote Guerini's summation of this medieval student of dentistry's rules for dental hygiene:

> "For the preservation of teeth—considered by him, quite rightly, a matter of great importance —Giovanni of Arcoli repeats the various counsels given on the subject by preceding writers, but he gives them as ten distinct canons or rules, creating in this way a kind of decalogue of dental hygiene. These rules are: (1) It is necessary to guard against the corruption of food and drink within the

stomach; therefore, easily corruptible food—milk, salt fish, etc.—must not be partaken of, and after meals all excessive movement, running exercises, bathing, coitus, and other causes that impair the digestion, must also be avoided. (2) Everything must be avoided that may provoke vomiting. (3) Sweet and viscous food—such as dried figs, preserves made with honey, etc.—must not be partaken of. (4) Hard things must not be broken with the teeth. (5) All food, drink, and other substances that set the teeth on edge must be avoided. (6) Food that is too hot or too cold must be avoided, and especially the rapid succession of hot and cold, and vice versa. (7) Leeks must not be eaten, as such a food, by its own nature, is injurious to the teeth. (8) The teeth must be cleaned at once, after every meal, from the particles of food left in them; and for this purpose thin pieces of wood should be used, somewhat broad at the ends, but not sharp-pointed or edged; and preference should be given to small cypress twigs, to the wood of aloes, or pine, rosemary, or juniper and similar sorts of wood which are rather bitter and styptic; care must, however, be taken not to search too long in the dental interstices and not to injure the gums or shake the teeth. (9) After this it is necessary to rinse the mouth by using by preference a vinous decoction of sage, or one of cinnamon, mastich, gallia, moschata, cubeb, juniper seeds, root of cyperus, and rosemary leaves. (10) The teeth must be rubbed with suitable dentrifices before going to bed, or else in the morning before breakfast. Although Avicenna recommended various oils for this purpose, Giovanni of Arcoli appears very hostile to

> oleaginous frictions, because he considers them very injurious to the stomach. He observes, besides, that whilst moderate frictions of brief duration are helpful to the teeth, strengthen the gums, prevent the formation of tartar, and sweeten the breath, too rough or too prolonged rubbing is, on the contrary, harmful to the teeth, and makes them liable to many diseases."

All this is so modern in many ways that we might expect a detailed exact knowledge of the anatomy of the teeth and even something of their embryology from Arculanus. It must not be forgotten, however, that coming as he does before the Renaissance, the medical sciences in the true sense of the word are as yet unborn. Men are accumulating information for practical purposes but not for the classification and co-ordination that was to make possible the scientific development of their knowledge.

Giovanni of Arcoli's acquaintance with the anatomy of the teeth was rather sadly lacking. He does not know even with certainty the number of roots that the teeth have. This has been attributed to the fact that he obtained most of his information from books, and had not the time to verify descriptions that he had found. It has been argued from this that he was himself probably not a practical dentist, and turned to that specialty only as a portion of his work as a general surgeon, and that consequently he was not sufficiently interested to verify his statements. His chapters on dentistry would seem to bear out this conclusion to some extent, though the very fact that one who was himself not specially interested in dental surgery should have succeeded in gathering together so much that anticipates modern ideas in dentistry, is of itself a proof of how much knowledge of the subject there was available for a serious student of that time. The anatomy of the teeth continued to be rather vague until about the middle of the next century when Eustachius, whose investigations of the anatomy of the head have deservedly brought him fame and the attachment of his name to the Eustachian canal, wrote his "Libellus de Dentibus—Manual of the Teeth," which is quite full, accurate, and detailed. Very little has been added to the microscopic anatomy of the teeth since Eustachius' time. He had the advantage, of course, of being intimately in contact with the great group of Renaissance anatomists,—Vesalius, Columbus, Varolius, Fallopius, and the others, the great fathers of anatomy. Besides, his position as Papal Physician and Professor of Anatomy at the Papal Medical School at Rome gave him opportunities for original investigation, such as were not easily obtained elsewhere.

Arculanus can scarcely be blamed, therefore, for not having anticipated the Renaissance, and we must take him as merely the culmination of medieval knowledge with regard to anatomy and surgery. Medieval medical men did not have the time nor apparently the incentive to make formal medical science, though it must not be forgotten, as has been said, that they did use the knowledge they obtained by their own and others' observation to excellent advantage for the practical benefit of ailing humanity. The sciences related to medicine are conscious developments that follow the evolution of practical medicine, nor must it be forgotten that far from always serving as an auxiliary to applied medical science, often indeed in the history of medicine scientific pursuits have led men away into side issues from which they had to be brought back by some genius medical observer. As might be expected, then, it is with regard to the practical treatment and general consideration of ailments of the teeth that Giovanni of Arcoli is most interesting. In this some of his chapters contain a marvellous series of surprises.

Arculanus was probably born towards the end of the fourteenth century. The date of his death is variously placed as either 1460 or 1484, with the probability in favor of the former. From 1412 to 1427 he was professor at Bologna, where in accordance with the non-specializing tendencies of the time he did not occupy a single chair but several in succession. He seems first to have taught Logic, then Moral Philosophy, and finally Medicine. His reputation in medicine drew many students to the university, and his fame spread all over Italy. The rival University of Padua then secured him, and he seems to have been for some twenty years there. Later apparently he accepted a professor's chair at Ferrara, where the D'Estes were trying to bring their university into prominence. It was at Ferrara that he died. He was a man of wide reading, of extensive experience, both of men and medicine, and one of the scholars of his time. His works are, as we have said, mainly excerpts from earlier writers and particularly the Arabians, but they contain enough of hints drawn from his own observation and experience to make his work of great value.

While, as Gurlt remarks in his "History of Surgery," Arculanus' name is one of those scarcely known—he is usually considered just one of many obscure writers of the end of the Middle Ages—his writings deserve a better fate. They contain much that is interesting and a great deal that must have been of the highest practical value to his contemporaries. They attracted wide attention in his own and immediately succeeding generations. The proof of this is that they exist in a large number of manuscript copies. Just as soon as printing was introduced his books appeared in edition after edition. His "Practica" was printed in no less than seven editions in Venice. Three of them appeared before the end of the fifteenth century, which places them among the *incunabula* of printing.

Probably nothing in the history of human intellectual interest is more striking than the excellent judgment displayed by the editors who selected the works to be printed at this time. Very few of them were trivial or insignificant. Fewer still were idle speculations, and most of them were almost of classical import for literature and science. Four editions of this work were printed in Venice in the sixteenth century, one of them as late as 1560, when the work done by such men as Vesalius, Columbus,

Eustachius, and Fallopius would seem to have made Arculanus out of date. The dates of the various editions are Venice, 1483, 1493, 1497, 1504, 1542, 1557, and 1560. Besides there was an edition printed at Basel in 1540.

Arculanus is said to have re-introduced the use of the seton, that is the method of producing intense counter-irritation by the introduction of some foreign body into an incision in the skin. We owe to him, too, according to Pagel in the chapters on medieval medicine in Puschmann's "Handbook of the History of Medicine," an excellent description of alcoholic insanity.

His directions for the treatment of conditions in the mouth and nose apart from the teeth are quite as explicit and practical, and in many ways quite as great an anticipation of some of our modern notions as what he has to say with regard to the teeth. For instance, in the treatment of polyps he says that they should be incised and cauterized. Soft polyps should be drawn out with a toothed tenaculum as far as can be without risk of breaking them off. The incision should be made at the root so that nothing or just as little as possible of the pathological structure be allowed to remain. It should be cut off with a fine scissors, or with a narrow file just small enough to permit its ingress into the nostrils, or with a scalpel without cutting edges on the sides, but only at its extremity, and this cutting edge should be broad and well sharpened. If there is danger of hemorrhage, or if there is fear of it, the instruments with which dissection is made should be fired (*igniantur*), that is, heated at least to a dull redness. Afterwards the stump, if any remains, should be touched with a hot iron or else with cauterizing agents so that as far as possible it should be obliterated.

After the operation a pledget of cotton dipped in the green ointment described by Rhazes should be placed in the nose. This pledget should have a string fastened to it, hanging from the nose in order that it may be easily removed. At times it may be necessary to touch the root of the polyp with a stylet on which cotton has been placed that has been dipped in *aqua fortis* (nitric acid). It is important that this cauterizing fluid should be rather strong so that after a certain number of touches a rather firm eschar is produced. In all these manipulations in the nose Arculanus recommends that the nose should be held well open by means of a nasal speculum. Pictures of all these instruments occur in his extant works, and indeed this constitutes one of their most interesting and valuable features. They are to be seen in Gurlt's "History of Surgery."

In some cases he had seen the polyp was so difficult to get at or was situated so far back in the nose that it could not be reached by means of a tenaculum or scissors, or even the special knife devised for that purpose. For these patients Arculanus describes an operation that is to be found in the older writers on surgery, Paul of Ægina

(Æginetus), Avicenna, and some of the other Arabian surgeons. For this three horse-tail hairs are twisted together and knotted in three or four places, and one end is passed through the nostrils and out through the mouth. The ends of this are then pulled on backward and forward after the fashion of a saw. Arculanus remarks evidently with the air of a man who has tried it and not been satisfied that this operation is quite uncertain, and seems to depend a great deal on chance, and much reliance must not be placed on it. Arculanus suggests a substitute method by which latent polyps or occult polyps as he calls them may be removed.

There is scarcely an important disease for which Arculanus has not some interesting suggestions, and the more one reads of him the more is one surprised to find how many things that we might think of as coming into the purview of medicine long after his time or at least as having been neglected from the time of the Greeks almost down to our own time are here treated explicitly, definitely, and with excellent practical suggestions. He has a good deal to say with regard to the treatment of angina, which he calls synanche, or synanchia, or cynanche, or angina. Parasynanche is a synonymous term, but refers to a milder synanche. He distinguished four forms of it. In one called canine angina, because the patient's tongue hangs out of his mouth, somewhat the same as from an overheated dog in the summer time, while at the same time the mouth is held open and he draws his breath pantingly, Arculanus suggests an unfavorable prognosis, and would seem to refer to those cases of Ludwig's angina in which there is involvement of the tongue and in which our prognosis continues to be of the very worst even to our own day. At times the angina causes such swelling in the throat that the breathing is interfered with completely. For this Arculanus' master, Rhazes, advised tracheotomy. Arculanus himself, however, apparently hesitated about that.

It is not surprising, then, to find that Arculanus is very explicit in his treatment of affections of the uvula. He divides its affections into *apostema,*]*ulcus, putredo sive corrosio, et casus. Apostema* was abscess, *ulcus* any rather deep erosion, *putredo* a gangrenous condition, and *casus* the fall of the uvula. This is the notorious falling of the soft palate which has always been in popular medical literature at least. Arculanus describes it as a preternatural elongation of the uvula which sometimes goes to such an extent as to make it resemble the tail of a mouse. For shorter elongations he suggests the cautery; for longer, excision followed by the cautery so that the greater portion of the extending part may be cut off. If people fear the knife he suggests following Rhazes, the application of an astringent powder directly to the part by blowing through a tube. His directions for the removal of the uvula are very definite. Seat the patient upon a stool in a bright light while an assistant holds the head; after the tongue has been firmly depressed by means of a speculum let the assistant hold this speculum in place. With the left hand then insert an instrument, a stilus, by which the uvula is pulled forward, and then remove the end of it by means of a heated knife or some other process of cauterization. The mouth should afterwards be washed out with fresh milk.

The application of a cauterizing solution by means of a cotton swab wrapped round the end of a sound may be of service in patients who refuse the actual cautery. To be successful the application must be firmly made and must be frequently repeated.

After this it is not surprising to find that Arculanus has very practical chapters on all the other ordinary surgical affections. Empyema is treated very thoroughly, liver abscess, ascites, which he warns must be emptied slowly, ileus especially when it reaches stercoraceous vomiting, and the various difficulties of urination, he divides them into dysuria, ischuria, and stranguria, are all discussed in quite modern fashion. He gives seven causes for difficulty of urination. One, some injury of the bladder; two, some lesion of the urethra; three, some pathological condition in the power to make the bladder contract; four, some injury of the muscle of the neck of the bladder; five, some pathological condition of the urine; six, some kidney trouble, and seven, some pathological condition of the general system. He takes up each one of these and discusses the various phases, causes, disposition, and predispositions that bring them about. One thing these men of the Middle Ages could do, they reasoned logically, they ordered what they had to say well, and they wrote it out straightforwardly.

That Arculanus' work with regard to dentistry was no mere chance and not solely theoretic can be understood very well from his predecessors, and that it formed a link in a continuous tradition which was well preserved we may judge from what is to be found in the writings of his great successor, Giovanni or John de Vigo, who is considered one of the great surgeons of the early Renaissance, and to whom we owe what is probably the earliest treatise on "Gun-shot Wounds." John of Vigo was a Papal physician and surgeon, generally considered one of the most distinguished members of the medical profession of his time. Two features of his writing on dental diseases deserve mention. He insists that abscesses of the gums shall be treated as other abscesses by being encouraged to come to maturity and then being opened. If they do not close promptly, an irritant Egyptian ointment containing verdigris and alum among other things should be applied to them. In the cure of old fistulous tracts near the teeth he employs not only this Egyptian ointment but also arsenic and corrosive sublimate. What he has to say with regard to the filling of the teeth is, however, most important. He says it with extreme brevity, but with the manner of a man thoroughly accustomed to doing it. "By means of a drill or file the putrefied or corroded part of the tooth should be completely removed. The cavity left should then be filled with gold leaf." It is evident that the members of the Papal court, the Cardinals and the Pope himself, had the advantage of rather good dentistry at John de Vigo's hands even as early as the beginning of the sixteenth century.

John de Vigo, however, is not medieval. He lived on into the sixteenth century and was influenced deeply by the Renaissance. He counts among the makers of modern medicine and surgery, as his authorship of the treatise on gun-shot wounds makes clear. He comes in a period that will be treated of in a later volume of this series on "Our Forefathers in Medicine."

XIII

CUSANUS AND THE FIRST SUGGESTION OF LABORATORY METHODS IN MEDICINE

As illustrating how, as we know more about the details of medical history, the beginnings of medical science and medical practice are pushed back farther and farther, a discussion in the *Berliner klinische Wochenschrift* a dozen years ago is of interest. Professor Ernest von Leyden, in sketching the history of the taking of the pulse as an important aid in diagnostics, said that John Floyer was usually referred to as the man who introduced the practice of determining the pulse rate by means of the watch. His work was done about the beginning of the eighteenth century. Professor von Leyden suggested, however, that William Harvey, the English physiologist, to whom is usually attributed the discovery of the circulation of the blood, had emphasized the value of the pulse in medical diagnosis, and also suggested the use of the watch in counting the pulse. Professor Carl Binz, of the University of Bonn, commenting on these remarks of Professor von Leyden, called attention to the fact that more than a century before the birth of either of these men, even the earlier, to whom the careful measurement of the pulse rate is thus attributed as a discovery, a distinguished German churchman, who died shortly after the middle of the fifteenth century, had suggested a method of accurate estimation of the pulse that deserves a place in medical history.

This suggestion is so much in accord with modern demands for greater accuracy in diagnosis that it seems not inappropriate to talk of it as the first definite attempt at laboratory methods in the department of medicine. The maker of the suggestion, curiously enough, was not a practising physician, but a mathematician and scholar, Cardinal Nicholas of Cusa, who is known in history as Cusanus from the Latin name of the town Cues on the Moselle River, some twenty-five miles south of Trèves, where he was born. His family name, Nicholas Krebs, has been entirely lost sight of in the name derived from his native town, which is the only reason why most of the world knows anything about that town. Cardinal Cusanus suggested that in various forms of disease and at various times of life, as in childhood, boyhood, manhood, and old age, the pulse was very different. It would be extremely valuable to have some method of accurately estimating, measuring, and recording these differences for medical purposes. At that time watches had not yet been invented, and it would have been very difficult to have estimated the time by the clocks, for almost the only clocks in existence were those in the towers of the cathedrals and of the public buildings. The first watches, Nuremberg eggs, as they were called, were not made by Peter Henlein until well on into the next century. The only method of measuring time with any accuracy in private houses was the clepsydra or water-clock, which measured the time intervals by the flow of a definite amount of water. Cardinal Cusanus suggested then that the water-clock should be employed for estimating the pulse frequency. His idea was that the amount of water which flowed while a hundred beats of the pulse were counted, should be weighed, and this weight compared with that of the average weight of water which flowed while a hundred beats of the normal pulse of a number of individuals of the same age and constitution were being counted.

This was a very single and a very ingenious suggestion. We have no means of knowing now whether it was adopted to any extent or not. It may seem rather surprising that a cardinal should have been the one to make such a suggestion. Cusanus, however, was very much interested in mathematics and in the natural sciences, and we have many wonderful suggestions from his pen. He was the first, for instance, to suggest, more than a century before Copernicus, that the earth was not the centre of the universe, and that it would not be absolutely at rest or, as he said, devoid of all motion. His words are: "*Terra igitur, quæ centrum esse nequit, motu omni carere non potest.*" He described very clearly how the earth moved round its own axis, and then he added, what cannot fail to be a surprising declaration for those in the modern times who think such an idea of much later origin, that he considered that the earth itself cannot be fixed, but moves as do the other stars in the heavens. The expression is so astonishing at that time in the world's history that it seems worth the while to give it in its original form, so that it may be seen clearly that it is not any subsequent far-fetched interpretation of his opinion, but the actual words themselves, that convey this idea. He said: "*Consideravi quod terra ista non potest esse fixa, sed movetur ut aliæ stellæ.*"

How clearly Cusanus anticipated another phase of our modern views may be judged from what he has to say in "De Docta Ignorantia" with regard to the constitution of the sun. It is all the more surprising that he should by some form of intuition reach such a conclusion, for the ordinary sources of information with regard to the sun would not suggest such an expression except to a genius, whose intuition outran by far the knowledge of his time.

The Cardinal said: "To a spectator on the surface of the sun the splendor which appears to us would be invisible, since it contains, as it were, an earth for its central mass, with a circumferential envelope of light and heat, and between the two an atmosphere of water and clouds and of ambient air." After reading that bit of precious astronomical science announced nearly five centuries ago, it is easy to understand how Copernicus could have anticipated other phases of our knowledge, as he did in his declarations that the figure of the earth is not a sphere, but is somewhat irregular, and that the orbit of the earth is not circular.

Cusanus was an extremely practical man, and was constantly looking for and devising methods of applying practical principles of science to ordinary life. As we shall see in discussing his suggestion for the estimation of the pulse rate later on, he made many other similar suggestions for diagnostic purposes in medicine, and set forth other applications of mathematics and mechanics to his generation.

Many of Cusanus' books have curiously modern names. He wrote, for instance, a series of mathematical treatises, in Latin of course, on "Geometric Transmutations," on "Arithmetical Complements," on "Mathematical Complements," on "Mathematical Perfection," and on "The Correction of the Calendar." In his time the calendar was in error by more than nine days, and Cusanus was one of those who aroused sufficient interest in the subject, so that in the next century the correction was actually made by the great Jesuit mathematician, Father Clavius. Perhaps the work of Cusanus that is best known is that "On Learned Ignorance—De Docta Ignorantia," in which the Cardinal points out how many things that educated people think they know are entirely wrong. It reminds one very much of Josh Billings's remark that it is not so much the ignorance of mankind that makes them ridiculous, as the knowing so many things that ain't so. It is from this work that the astronomical quotations which we have made are taken. The book that is of special interest to physicians is his dialogue "On Static Experiments," which he wrote in 1450, and which contains the following passages:

> "Since the weight of the blood and the urine of a healthy and of a diseased man, of a young man and an old man, of a German and an African, is different for each individual, why would it not be a great benefit to the physician to have all of these various differences classified? For I think that a physician would make a truer judgment from the weight of the urine viewed in connection with its color than he could make from its color alone, which might be fallacious. So, also, weight might be used as a means of identifying the roots, the stems, the leaves, the fruits, the seeds, and the juice of plants if the various weights of all the plants were properly noted, together with their variety, according to locality. In this way the physician would appreciate their nature better by means of their weight than if he

judged them by their taste alone. He might know, then, from a comparison of the weights of the plants and their various parts when compared with the weight of the blood and the urine, how to make an application and a dosage of drugs from the concordances and differences of the medicaments, and even might be able to make an excellent prognosis in the same way. Thus, from static experiments, he would approach by a more precise knowledge to every kind of information.

"Do you not think if you would permit the water from the narrow opening of a clepsydra [water-clock] to flow into a basin for as long as was necessary to count the pulse a hundred times in a healthy young man, and then do the same thing for an ailing young man, that there would be a noticeable difference between the weights of the water that would flow during the period? From the weight of the water, therefore, one would arrive at a better knowledge of the differences in the pulse of the young and the old, the healthy and the unhealthy, and so, also, as to information with regard to various diseases, since there would be one weight and, therefore, one pulse in one disease, and another weight and another pulse in another disease. In this way a better judgment of the differences in the pulse could be obtained than from the touch of the vein, just as more can be known from the urine about its weight than from its color alone.

"Just in the same way would it not be possible to make a more accurate judgment with regard to the breathing, if the inspirations and expirations were studied according to the

> weight of the water that passed during a certain interval? If, while water was flowing from a clepsydra, one were to count a hundred expirations in a boy, and then in an old man, of course, there would not be the same amount of water at the end of the enumeration. Then this same thing might be done for other ages and states of the body. As a consequence, when the physician once knew what the weight of water that represented the number of expirations of a healthy boy or youth, and then of an individual of the same age ill of some infirmity or other, there is no doubt that, by this observation, he will come to a knowledge of the health or illness and something about the case, and, perhaps, also with more certainty would be able to choose the remedy and the dose required. If he found in a healthy young man apparently the same weight as in an old and decrepit individual, he might readily be brought to the conclusion that the young man would surely die, and in this way have some evidence for his prognosis in the case. Besides, if in fevers, in the same way, careful studies were made of the differences in the weight of water for pulse and respiration in the warm and the cold paroxysms, would it not be possible thus to know the disease better and, perhaps, also get a more efficacious remedy?"

As will be seen from this passage, Cusanus had many more ideas than merely the accurate estimation of the pulse frequency when he suggested the use of the water-clock. Evidently the thought had come to him that the specific gravity of the substances, that is, their weight in comparison to the weight of water, might be valuable information.Before his time, physicians had depended only on the color and the taste of the urine for diagnostic purposes. He proposed that they should weigh it, and even suggested that they should weigh, also, the blood, I suppose in case of venesection, for comparison's sake. He also thought that the comparative weight of various roots, stems, leaves, juices of plants might give hints for the therapeutic uses of these substances. This is the sort of idea that we are apt to think of as typically modern. Specific gravities and atomic weights have been more than once supposed to represent laws in therapeutics, which so far, however, we have not succeeded in finding, but it is interesting to realize that it is nearly five hundred years since the first thought in this line was clearly expressed by a distinguished thinker and scientific writer.

There are many interesting expressions in Cusanus' writings which contradict most of the impressions commonly entertained with regard to the scholars of the Middle Ages. It is usually assumed that they did not think seriously, but speculatively, that they feared to think for themselves, neglected the study of nature around them, considered authority the important source of knowledge, and were as far as possible from the standpoint of modern scientific students and investigators. Here is a passage from Nicholas, on knowing and thinking, that might well have been written by a great intellectual man at any time in the world's history, and that could only emanate from a profound scholar at any time.

"To know and to think, to see the truth with the eye of the mind, is always a joy. The older a man grows the greater is the pleasure which it affords him, and the more he devotes himself to the search after truth, the stronger grows his desire of possessing it. As love is the life of the heart, so is the endeavor after knowledge and truth the life of the mind. In the midst of the movements of time, of the daily work of life, of its perplexities and contradictions, we should lift our gaze fearlessly to the clear vault of heaven, and seek ever to obtain a firmer grasp of and a keener insight into the origin of all goodness and beauty, the capacities of our own hearts and minds, the intellectual fruits of mankind throughout the centuries, and the wondrous works of nature around us; at the same time remembering always that in humility alone lies true greatness, and that knowledge and wisdom are alone profitable in so far as our lives are governed by them."

The career of Nicholas of Cusa is interesting, because it sums up so many movements, and, above all, educational currents in the fifteenth century. He was born in the first year of the century, and lived to be sixty-four. He was the son of a wine grower, and attracted the attention of his teachers because of his intellectual qualities. In spite of comparatively straitened circumstances, then, he was afforded the best opportunities of the time for education. He went first to the school of the Brethren of the Common Life at Deventer, the intellectual cradle of so many of the scholars of this century. Such men as Erasmus, Conrad Mutianus, Johann Sintheim, Hermann von dem Busche, whom Strauss calls "the missionary of human wisdom," and the teacher of most of these, Alexander Hegius, who has been termed the schoolmaster of Germany, with Nicholas of Cusa and Rudolph Agricola and others, who might readily be mentioned, are the fruits of the teaching of these schools of the Brethren of the Common Life, in one of which Thomas à Kempis, the author of "The

Imitation of Christ," was, for seventy years out of his long life of ninety, a teacher.

Cusanus succeeded so well at school that he was later sent to the University of Heidelberg, and subsequently to Padua, where he took up the study of Roman law, receiving his doctorate at the age of twenty-three. This series of educational opportunities will be surprising only to those who do not know educational realities at the beginning of the fifteenth century. There has never been a time when a serious seeker after knowledge could find more inspiration. On his return to Germany, Father Krebs became canon of the cathedral in Coblenz. This gave him a modest income, and leisure for intellectual work which was eagerly employed. He was scarcely more than thirty when he was chosen as a delegate to the Council at Basel. After this he was made Archdeacon of the Cathedral of Lüttich, and from this time his rise in ecclesiastical preferment was rapid. He had attracted so much attention at the Council of Basel that he was chosen as a legate of the Pope for the bringing about certain reforms in Germany. Subsequently he was sent on ecclesiastical missions to the Netherlands, and even to Constantinople. At the early age of forty he was made a Cardinal. After this he was always considered as one of the most important consultors of the Papacy in all matters relating to Germany. During the last twenty-five years of his life in all the relations of the Holy See to Germany, appeal was constantly made to the wisdom, the experience, and the thoroughly conservative, yet foreseeing, judgment of this son of the people, whose education had lifted him up to be one of the leaders of men in Europe.

It was during this time that he wrote most of his books on mathematics, which have earned for him a prominent place in Cantor's "History of Mathematics," about a score of pages being devoted to his work. Much of his thinking was done while riding on horseback or in the rude vehicles of the day on the missions to which he was sent as Papal Legate. He is said to have worked out the formula for the cycloid curve while watching the path described by flies that had lighted on the wheels of his carriage, and were carried forward and around by them. His scientific books, though they included such startling anticipations of Copernicus' doctrines as we have already quoted (Copernicus did not publish the first sketch of his theory for more than a quarter of a century after Cusanus' death), far from disturbing his ecclesiastical advancement or injuring his career as a churchman, seem actually to have been considered as additional reasons for considering him worthy of confidence and consultation.

As the result of his careful studies of conditions in Germany, he realized very clearly how much of unfortunate influence the political status of the German people, with their many petty rulers and the hampering of development consequent upon the trivial rivalries, the constant bickerings, and the inordinate jealousies of these numerous princelings, had upon his native country. Accordingly, towards the end of his life he sketched what he thought would be the ideal political status for the German people. As in everything that he wrote, he went straight to the heart of the matter and, without mincing words, stated just exactly what he thought ought to be done. Considering that this scheme of Cusanus for the prosperity and right government of the German people was not accomplished until more than four centuries after his death, it is interesting, indeed, to realize how this clergyman of the middle of the fifteenth century should have come to any such thought. Nothing, however, makes it clearer than this, that it is not time that fosters thinking, but that great men at any time come to great thoughts. Cusanus wrote:

> "The law and the kingdom should be placed under the protection of a single ruler or authority. The small separate governments of princes and counts consume a disproportionately large amount of revenue without furnishing any real security. For this reason we must have a single government, and for its support we must have a definite amount of the income from taxes and revenues yearly set aside by a representative parliament and before this parliament (reichstag) must be given every year a definite account of the money that was spent during the preceding year."

Cusanus' life and work stand, then, as a type of the accomplishment, the opportunities, the power of thought, the practical scholarship, the mathematical accuracy, the fine scientific foresight of a scholar of the fifteenth century. For us, in medicine, it is interesting indeed to realize that it is from a man of this kind that a great new departure in medicine with regard to the employment of exact methods of diagnosis had its first suggestion in modern times. The origin of that suggestion is typical. It has practically always been true that it was not the man who had exhausted, or thought that he had done so, all previous medical knowledge, who made advances in medicine for us. It has nearly always been a young man early in his career, and at a time when, as yet, his mind was not overloaded with the medical theories of his own time. Cusanus was probably not more than thirty when he made the suggestion which represents the first practical hint for the use of laboratory methods in modern medicine. It came out of his thoughtful consideration of medical problems rather than from a store of garnered information as to what others thought. It is a lesson in the precious value of breadth of education and serious training of mind for real progress at all times.

XIV

BASIL VALENTINE, LAST OF THE ALCHEMISTS, FIRST OF THE CHEMISTS

> "Fieri enim potest ut operator erret et a via regia deflectat, sed ut erret natura quando recte tractatur fieri non potest."

> "For it is quite possible that the physician should err and be turned aside from the straight (royal) road, but that nature when she

> is rightly treated should err is quite impossible."

This is one of the preliminary maxims of a treatise on medicine written by a physician born not later than the first half of the fifteenth century, and who may have lived even somewhat earlier. We are so prone to think of the men of that time as utterly dependent on authority, not daring to follow their own observation, suspecting nature, and almost sure to be convinced that only by going counter to her could success in the treatment of disease be obtained, that it is a surprise to most people to find how completely the attitude of mind, that is supposed to be so typically modern in this regard, was anticipated full four centuries ago. There are other expressions of this same great physician and medical writer, Basil Valentine, which serve to show how faithfully he strove with the lights that he had to work out the treatment of patients, just as we do now, by trying to find out nature's way, so as to imitate her beneficent processes and purposes. It is quite clear that he is but one of many faithful, patient observers and experimenters—true scientists in the best sense of the word—who lived in all the centuries of the Middle Ages. Speculations and experiments with regard to the elixir of life, the philosopher's stone, and the transmutation of metals, are presumed to have filled up all the serious interests of the alchemists, supposed to be almost the only scientists of those days. As a matter of fact, however, men were making original observations of profound significance, and these were considered so valuable by their contemporaries that, though printing had not yet been invented, even the immense labor involved in the manifold copying of large folio volumes by the slow hand process did not suffice to deter them from multiplying the writings of these men so numerously that they were preserved in many copies for future generations, until the printing press came to perpetuate them.

Of this there is abundant evidence in the preceding pages as regards medicine, and, above all, surgery, while a summary of accomplishments of workers in other departments will be found in Appendix II, "Science at the Medieval Universities."

At the beginning of the twentieth century, with some of the supposed foundations of modern chemistry crumbling to pieces under the influence of the peculiarly active light thrown upon our nineteenth century chemical theories by the discovery of radium, and our observations on radio-active elements generally, there is a reawakening of interest in some of the old-time chemical observers, whose work used to be laughed at as so unscientific, or, at most, but a caricature of real science, and whose theory of the transmutation of elements into one another was considered so absurd. It is interesting in the light of this to recall that the idea that the elementary substances were essentially distinct from each other, and that it would be impossible under any circumstances to convert one element into another, belongs entirely to the nineteenth century. Even so deeply scientific a mind as that of Newton, in the preceding century, could not bring itself to acknowledge the tradition, that came to be accepted subsequent to his time, of the absurdity of metallic transformation. On the contrary, he believed quite formally in transmutation as a basic chemical principle, and declared that it might be expected to occur at any time. He had seen specimens of gold ores in connection with metallic copper, and concluded that this was a manifestation of the natural transformation of one of these yellow metals into the other.

With the discovery that radium transforms itself into helium, and that, indeed, all the so-called radioactivities of the heavy metals are probably due to a natural transmutation process constantly at work, the ideas of the older chemists cease entirely to be a subject for amusement. The physical chemists of the present day are very ready to admit that the old teaching of the absolute independence of something over seventy elements is no longer tenable, except as a working hypothesis. The doctrine of "matter and form," taught for so many centuries by the scholastic philosophers, which proclaimed that all matter is composed of two principles, an underlying material substratum, and a dynamic or informing principle, has now more acknowledged verisimilitude, or lies at least closer to the generally accepted ideas of the most progressive scientists, than it has at any time for the last two or three centuries. Not only the great physicists, but also the great chemists, are speculating along lines that suggest the existence of but one form of matter, modified according to the energies that it possesses under a varying physical and chemical environment. This is, after all, only a restatement in modern times of the teaching of St. Thomas of Aquin, in the thirteenth century.

It is not surprising, then, that there should be a reawakening of interest in the lives of some of the men, who, dominated by some of the earlier scholastic ideas, by the tradition of the possibility of finding the philosopher's stone, which would transmute the baser metals into the precious metals, devoted themselves with quite as much zeal as any modern chemist to the observation of chemical phenomena. One of the most interesting of these—indeed, he might well be said to be the greatest of the alchemists—is the man whose only name that we know is that which appears on a series of manuscripts written in the High German dialect of the end of the fifteenth and the beginning of the sixteenth century. That name is Basil Valentine, and the writer, according to the best historical traditions, was a Benedictine monk. The name Basil Valentine may only have been a pseudonym, for it has been impossible to trace it among the records of the monasteries of the time. That the writer was a monk, however, there seems to be no room for doubt, for his writings give abundant evidence of it, and, besides, in printed form they began to have their vogue at a time when there was little likelihood of their being attributed to a monastic source, unless an indubitable tradition connected them with some monastery.

This Basil Valentine (to accept the only name we have) did so much for the science of the composition of substances that he eminently deserves the designation that has been given him of the last of the alchemists and the first of the chemists. There is practically a universal recognition of the fact now that he deserves also the title of the Founder of Pharmaceutical Chemistry, not only because of the value of the observations contained in his writings, but also because of the fact that they proved so suggestive to certain scientific geniuses during the century succeeding Valentine's life. Almost more than to have added to the precious heritage of knowledge for mankind, it is a boon for a scientific observer to have awakened the spirit of observation in others, and to be the founder of a new school of thought. This Basil Valentine undoubtedly did, and, in the Renaissance, the incentive from his writings for such men as Paracelsus is easy to appreciate.

Besides, his work furnishes evidence that the investigating spirit was abroad just when it is usually supposed not to have been, for the Thuringian monk surely did not do all his investigation alone, but must have owed, as well as given, many a suggestion to his contemporaries.

Some ten years ago, when Sir Michael Foster, professor of physiology in the University of Cambridge, England, was invited to deliver the Lane Lectures at the Cooper Medical

College in San Francisco, he took for his subject "The History of Physiology." In the course of his lecture on "The Rise of Chemical Physiology" he began with the name of Basil Valentine, who first attracted men's attention to the many chemical substances around them that might be used in the treatment of disease, and said of him:

> "He was one of the alchemists, but in addition to his inquiries into the properties of metals and his search for the philosopher's stone, he busied himself with the nature of drugs, vegetable and mineral, and with their action as remedies for disease. He was no anatomist, no physiologist, but rather what nowadays we should call a pharmacologist. He did not care for the problem of the body, all he sought to understand was how the constituents of the soil and of plants might be treated so as to be available for healing the sick and how they produced their effects. We apparently owe to him the introduction of many chemical substances, for instance of hydrochloric acid, which he prepared from oil and vitriol of salt, and of many vegetable drugs. And he was apparently the author of certain conceptions which, as we shall see, played an important part in the development of chemistry and of physiology. To him, it seems, we owe the idea of the three 'elements,' as they were and have been called, replacing the old idea of the ancients of the four elements—earth, air, fire, and water. It must be remembered, however, that both in the ancient and the new idea the word 'element' was not intended to mean that which it means to us now, a fundamental unit of matter, but a general quality or property of

> matter. The three elements of Valentine were: (1) sulphur, or that which is combustible, which is changed or destroyed, or which at all events disappears during burning or combustion; (2) mercury, that which temporarily disappears during burning or combustion, which is dissociated in the burning from the body burnt, but which may be recovered, that is to say, that which is volatile, and (3) salt, that which is fixed, the residue or ash which remains after burning."

It is a little bit hard in our time for most people to understand just how such a development of thoroughly scientific chemical notions, with investigations for their practical application, should have come before the end of the Middle Ages. This difficulty of understanding, however, we are coming to realize in recent years, is entirely due to our ignorance of the period. We have known little or nothing about the science of the Middle Ages, because it was hidden away in rare old books, in rather difficult Latin, not easy to get at, and still less easy to understand always, and we have been prone to conclude that since we knew nothing about it, there must have been nothing. Just inasmuch as we have learned something definite about the medieval scholars, our admiration has increased. Professor Clifford Allbutt, the Regius Professor of Medicine at the University of Cambridge, in his Harveian Oration, delivered before the Royal College of Physicians in 1900, on "Science and Medieval Thought" (London, 1901), declared that "the schoolmen, in digging for treasure, cultivated the field of knowledge even for Galileo and Harvey, for Newton and Darwin." He might have added that they had laid foundations in all our modern sciences, in chemistry quite as well as in astronomy, physiology, and the medical sciences, in mathematics and botany.

In chemistry the advances made during the thirteenth, fourteenth, and fifteenth centuries were, perhaps, even more noteworthy than those in any other department of science. Albertus Magnus, who taught at Paris, wrote no less than sixteen treatises on chemical subjects, and, notwithstanding the fact that he was a theologian as well as a scientist, and that his printed works fill some *fifteen folio volumes,* he somehow found the time to make many observations for himself, and performed numberless experiments in order to clear up doubts. The larger histories of chemistry accord him his proper place, and hail him as a great founder in chemistry, and a pioneer in original investigation.

Even St. Thomas of Aquin, much as he was occupied with theology and philosophy, found some time to devote to chemical questions. After all, this is only what might have been expected of the favorite pupil of Albertus Magnus. Three treatises on chemical subjects from Aquinas' pen have been preserved for us, and it is to him that we are said to owe the use, in the Western world at least, of the word amalgam, which he first employed in describing various chemical methods of metallic combination with mercury that were discovered in the search for the genuine transmutation of metals.

Albertus Magnus' other great scientific pupil, Roger Bacon, the English Franciscan friar, followed more closely in the scientific ways of his great master, devoting himself almost entirely to the physical sciences. Altogether he wrote some eighteen treatises on chemical subjects. For a long time it was considered that he was the inventor of gunpowder, though this is now known to have been introduced into Europe by the Arabs. Roger Bacon studied gunpowder and various other explosive combinations in considerable detail, and it is for this reason that he obtained the undeserved reputation of being an original discoverer in this line. How well he realized how much might be accomplished by means of the energy stored up in explosives, can, perhaps, be best appreciated from the fact that he suggested that boats would go along the rivers and across seas without either sails or oars, and that carriages would go along the streets without horse or man power. He considered that man would eventually invent a method of harnessing these explosive mixtures, and of utilizing their energies for his purposes without danger. It is curiously interesting to find, as we begin the twentieth century, and gasolene is so commonly used for the driving of automobiles and motor boats, and is being introduced even into heavier transportation as the most available source of energy for suburban traffic, at least, that this generation should only be fulfilling the idea of the old Franciscan friar of the thirteenth century, who prophesied that in explosives there was the secret of eventually manageable energy for transportation purposes.

Succeeding centuries were not as fruitful in great scientists as the thirteenth, and yet, in the second half of the thirteenth, there was a Pope, John XXI,who had been a physician and professor of medicine before his election to the Papacy, three of whose scientific treatises—one on the transmutation of metals, which he considers an impossibility, at least as far as the manufacture of gold and silver was concerned; a treatise on diseases of the eyes, to which good authorities have not hesitated to give lavish praise for its practical value, considering the conditions in which it was written; and, finally, his treatise on the preservation of the health, written when he was himself over eighty years of age—are all considered by good authorities as worthy of the best scientific spirit of the time.

During the fourteenth century, Arnold of Villanova, the inventor of nitric acid, and the two Hollanduses, kept up the tradition of original investigation in chemistry. Altogether there are some dozen treatises from these three men on chemical subjects. The Hollanduses particularly did their work in a spirit of thoroughly frank, original investigation. They were more interested in minerals than in any other class of substances, but did not waste much time on the question of transmutation of metals. Professor Thompson, the professor of chemistry at Edinburgh, said, in his "History of Chemistry," many years ago, that the Hollanduses give very clear descriptions of their processes of treating minerals in investigating their composition, and these serve to show that their knowledge was by no means entirely theoretical, or acquired only from books.

It is not surprising, then, to have a great investigating pharmacologist come along sometime about the beginning of the fifteenth century, when, according to the best authorities, Basil Valentine was born. From traditions he seems to have had a rather long life, and his years run nearly parallel with his century. His career is a typical example of the personally obscure and intellectually brilliant lives which the old monks lived. Probably in nothing have recent generations been more deceived in historical matters than in their estimation of the intellectual attainments and accomplishment of the old monks. The more that we know of them, not from second-hand authorities, but from their own books and from what they accomplished in art and architecture, in agriculture, in science of all kinds, the more do we realize what busy men they were, and appreciate what genius they often brought to the solution of great problems. We have had much negative pseudo-information brought together with the definite purpose of discrediting monasticism, and now that positive information is gradually being accumulated, it is almost a shock to find how different are the realities of the story of the intellectual life during the Middle Ages from what many writers had pictured them.

To those who may be surprised that a man who did great things in medicine should have lived during the fifteenth century, it may be well to recall the names and a little of the accomplishment of the men of this period, who were Basil Valentine's contemporaries, at least in the sense that some portion of their lives and influence was coeval with his. Before the end of this century Columbus had discovered America, and by no happy accident, for many men of his generation did correspondingly great work. Cardinal Nicholas of Cusa had developed mathematics and applied mathematical ideas to the heavens, so that he could announce the conclusion that the earth was a star, like the other stars, and moved in the heavens as they do. Contemporary with Cusanus was Regiomontanus, who has been proclaimed the father of modern astronomy, and a distinguished mathematician. Toscanelli, the Florentine astronomer, whose years run almost parallel with those of the fifteenth century, did fine scholarly work, which deeply influenced Columbus and the great navigators of the time. The universities in Italy were attracting students from all over Europe, and such men as Linacre and Dr. Caius went down there from England. Raphael was but a young man at the end of the century, but he had done some noteworthy painting before it closed. Leonardo da Vinci was born just about the middle of the century, and did some marvellous work before the end of that century. Michael Angelo was only twenty-five at the close of the century, but he, too, did fine work, even at this early age.

Among the other great Italian painters of this century are Fra Angelico, Perugino, Raphael's master, Pinturicchio, Signorelli, the pupil of his uncle, Vasari, almost as distinguished, Botticelli, Titian, and very many others, who would have been famous leaders in art in any other but this supremely great period.

It was not only in Italy, however, that there was a wonderful outburst of genius at this time, for Germany also saw the rise of a number of great men during this period. Jacob Wimpheling, the "Schoolmaster of Germany," as he has been called, whose educational work did much to determine the character of German education for two centuries, was born in 1450. Rudolph Agricola, who influenced the intellectual Europe of this time deeply, was born in 1443. Erasmus, one of the greatest of scholars, of teachers, and of controversialists, was born in 1467. Johann Reuchlin, the great linguist, who, next to Erasmus, is the most important character in the German Renaissance, was born in 1455. Then there was Sebastian Brant, the author of "The Ship of Fools," and Alexander Hegius, both of this same period. The most influential of them all, Thomas à Kempis, who died in 1471, and whose little book, "The Following of Christ," has influenced every generation deeply ever since, was probably a close contemporary of Basil Valentine. When one knows what European, and especially German scholars, were accomplishing at this time, no room is left for surprise that Basil Valentine should have lived and done work in medicine at this period that was to influence deeply the after history of medicine.

Most of what Basil Valentine did was accomplished in the first half of the fifteenth century. Coming, as he did, before the invention of printing, when the spirit of tradition was more rife and dominating than it has been since, it is almost needless to say that there are many curious legends associated with his name. Two centuries before his time, Roger Bacon, doing his work in England, had succeeded in attracting so much attention even from the common people, because of his wonderful scientific discoveries, that his name became a byword, and many strange magical feats were attributed to him. Friar Bacon was the great wizard, even in the plays of the Elizabethan period. A number of the same sort of myths attached themselves to the Benedictine monk of the fifteenth century. He was proclaimed in popular story to have been a wonderful magician. Even his manuscript, it was said, had not been published directly, but had been hidden in a pillar in the church attached to his monastery, and had been discovered there after the splitting open of the pillar by a bolt of lightning from heaven. It is the extension of this tradition that has sometimes led to the assumption that Valentine lived in an earlier century, some even going so far as to say that he, too, like Roger Bacon, was a product of the thirteenth century. It seems reasonably possible, however, to separate the traditional from what is actual in his existence, and thus to obtain some idea at least of his work, if not of the details of his life. The internal evidence from his works enables the historian of science to place his writing within half a century of the discovery of America.

One of the myths that have gathered around the name of Basil Valentine, because it has become a commonplace in philology, has probably made him more generally known than any of his actual discoveries. In one of the most popular of the old-fashioned text-books of chemistry in use about half a century ago, in the chapter on antimony, there was a story that students, if I may judge from my own experience, never forgot. It was said that Basil Valentine, a monk of the Middle Ages, was the discoverer of this substance. After having experimented with it in a number of ways, he threw some of it out of his laboratory one day when the swine of the monastery, finding it, proceeded to gobble it up, together with some other refuse. Just when they were finishing it, the monk discovered what they were doing. He feared the worst from it, but took the occasion to observe the effect upon the swine very carefully. He found that, after a preliminary period of digestive disturbance, these swine developed an enormous appetite, and became fatter than any of the others. This seemed a rather desirable result, and Basil Valentine, ever on the search for the practical, thought that he might use the remedy to good purpose on the members of the community. Some of the monks in the monastery were of rather frail health and delicate constitution, and most of them were rather thin, and he thought that the putting on of a little fat, provided it could be accomplished without infringement of the rule, might be a good thing for them. Accordingly, he administered, surreptitiously, some of the salts of antimony, with which he was experimenting, in the food served to these monks. The result, however, was not so favorable as in the case of the hogs. Indeed, according to one, though less authentic, version of the story, some of the poor monks, the unconscious subjects of the experiment, perished as the result of the ingestion of the antimonial compounds. According to the better version, they suffered only the usual unpleasant consequences of taking antimony, which are, however, quite enough for a fitting climax to the story. Basil Valentine called the new substance which he had discovered antimony, that is, *opposed to monks*. It might be good for hogs, but it was a form of monks' bane, as it were.[30]

Unfortunately for most of the good stories of history, modern criticism has nearly always failed to find any authentic basis for them, and they have had to go the way of the legends of Washington's hatchet and Tell's apple. We are sorry to say that that seems to be true also of this particular story. Antimony, the word, is very probably derived from certain dialectic forms of the Greek word for the metal, and the name is no more derived from *anti* and *monachus* than it is from *anti* and *monos* (opposed to single existence), another fictitious derivation that has been suggested, and one whose etymological value is supposed to consist in the fact that antimony is practically never found alone in nature.

Notwithstanding the apparent cloud of unfounded traditions that are associated with his name, there can be no doubt at all of the fact that Valentinus—to give him the Latin name by which he is commonly designated in foreign literatures—was one of the great geniuses, who, working in obscurity, make precious steps into the unknown that enable humanity after them to see things more clearly than ever before. There are definite historical grounds for placing Basil Valentine as the first of the series of careful observers who differentiated chemistry from the old alchemy and applied its precious treasures of information to the uses of medicine. It is said to have been because of the study of Basil Valentine's work that Paracelsus broke away from the Galenic traditions, so supreme in medicine up to his time, and began our modern pharmaceutics. Following Paracelsus came Van Helmont, the father of modern medical chemistry, and these three did more than any others to enlarge the scope of medication and to make observation rather than authority the most important criterion of truth in medicine. Indeed, the work of this trio of men of the fifteenth and sixteenth centuries—the Renaissance in medicine as in art—dominated medical treatment, or at least the department of pharmaceutics, down almost to our own day, and their influence is still felt in drug-giving.

While we do not know the absolute data of either the birth or the death of Basil Valentine and are not sure of the exact period even in which he lived and did his work, we are sure that a great original observer about the time of the invention of printing studied mercury and sulphur and various salts of the metals, and above all introduced antimony to the notice of the scientific world, and especially to the favor of practitioners of medicine. His book, "The Triumphal Chariot of Antimony," is full of conclusions not quite justified by his premises nor by his observations. There is no doubt, however, that the observational method which he employed furnished an immense amount of knowledge, and formed the basis of the method of investigation by which the chemical side of medicine was to develop during the next two or three centuries. Great harm was done by the abuse of antimony, but then great harm is done by the abuse of anything, no matter how good it may be. For a time it came to be the most important drug in medicine and was only replaced by venesection.

The fact of the matter is that doctors were looking for effects from their drugs, and antimony is, above all things, effective. Patients, too, wished to see the effect of the medicines they took. They do so even yet, and when antimony was administered there was no doubt about its working.

The most interesting of Basil Valentine's books, and the one which has had the most enduring influence, is undoubtedly "The Triumphal Chariot of Antimony."[31]

It has been translated and has had a wide vogue in every language of modern Europe. Its recommendation of antimony had such an effect upon medical practice that it continued to be the most important drug in the pharmacopœia down almost to the middle of the nineteenth century. If any proof were needed that Basil Valentine or that the author of the books that go under the name was a monk it would be found in the introduction to this volume, which not only states that fact very clearly, but also in doing so makes use of language that shows the writer to have been deeply imbued with the old monastic spirit. I quote the first paragraph of this introduction because it emphasizes this. The quotation is taken from the English translation of the work as published in London in 1678. Curiously enough, seeing the obscurity surrounding Valentine himself, we do not know for sure who made the translation. The translator apologizes somewhat for the deeply religious spirit of the book, but considers that he was not justified in eliminating any of this. The paragraph is left in the quaint, old-fashioned form so eminently suited to the thoughts of the old master, and the spelling and use of capitals is not changed.

> "Basil Valentine: His Triumphant Chariot of Antimony.—Since I, Basil Valentine, by Religious Vows am bound to live according to

the order of St. Benedict and that requires another manner of Spirit of Holiness than the common state of Mortals exercised in the profane business of this World; I thought it my duty before all things, in the beginning of this little book, to declare what is necessary to be known by the pious Spagyrist [old-time name for medical chemist], inflamed with an ardent desire of this Art, as what he ought to do, and whereunto to direct his striving, that he may lay such foundations of the whole matter as may be stable; lest his Building, shaken with the Winds, happen to fall, and the whole Edifice to be involved in shameful Ruine which otherwise being founded on more firm and solid principles, might have continued for a long series of time. Which Admonition I judged was, is and always will be a necessary part of my religious Office; especially since we must all die, and no one of us which are now, whether high or low, shall long be seen among the number of men. For it concerns me to recommend these Meditations of Mortality to Posterity, leaving them behind me, not only that honor may be given to the Divine Majesty, but also that men may obey him sincerely in all things.

"In this my meditation I found that there were five principal heads, chiefly to be considered by the wise and prudent spectators of our Wisdom and Art. The first of which is Invocation of God. The second, Contemplation of Nature. The third, True Preparation. The fourth, the Way of Using. The fifth, Utility and Fruit. For he who regards not these, shall never obtain place among true Chymists, or fill up the number of perfect Spagyrists.

> Therefore, touching these five heads, we shall here following treat and so far declare them, as that the general Work may be brought to light and perfected by an intent and studious Operator."

This book, though the title might seem to indicate it, is not devoted entirely to the study of antimony, but contains many important additions to the chemistry of the time. For instance, Basil Valentine explains in this work how what he calls the spirit of salt might be obtained. He succeeded in manufacturing this material by treating common salt with oil of vitriol and heat. From the description of the uses to which he put the end product of his chemical manipulation, it is evident that under the name of spirit of salt he is describing what we now know as hydrochloric acid. This is said to be the first definite mention of it in the history of science, and the method suggested for its preparation is not very different from that employed even at the present time. He also suggests in his volume how alcohol may be obtained in high strengths. He distilled the spirit obtained from wine over carbonate of potassium, and thus succeeded in depriving it of a great proportion of its water. We have said that he was deeply interested in the philosopher's stone. Naturally this turned his attention to the study of metals, and so it is not surprising to find that he succeeded in formulating a method by which metallic copper could be obtained. The material used for the purpose was copper pyrites, which was changed to an impure sulphate of copper by the action of oil of vitriol and moist air. The sulphate of copper occurred in solution, and the copper could be precipitated from it by plunging an iron bar into it. Basil Valentine recognized the presence of this peculiar yellow metal, and studied some of its qualities. He does not seem to have been quite sure, however, whether the phenomenon that he witnessed was not really a transmutation of at least some of the iron into copper as a consequence of the other chemicals present. There are some observations on chemical physiology, and especially with regard to respiration, in the book on antimony which show their author to have anticipated the true explanation of the theory of respiration. He states that animals breathe because air is needed to support their life, and that all the animals exhibit the phenomenon of respiration. He even insists that the fishes, though living in water, breathe air, and he adduces in support of this idea the fact that whenever a river is entirely frozen the fishes die. The reason for this being, according to this old-time physiological chemist, not that the fishes are frozen to death, but that they are not able to obtain air in the ice as they did in the water, and consequently perish.

There are many testimonials to the practical character of all his knowledge and his desire to apply it for the benefit of humanity. The old monk could not repress the expression of his impatience with physicians who gave to patients for "diseases of which they knew little, remedies of which they knew less." For him it was an unpardonable sin for a physician not to have faithfully studied the various mixtures that he prescribed for his patients, and not to know not only their appearance and taste and effect, but also the limits of their application. Considering that at the present time it is a frequent source of complaint that physicians often prescribe remedies with even whose physical appearance they are not familiar and whose composition is often quite unknown to them, this complaint of the old-time chemist alchemist will be all the more interesting for the modern physician. It is evident that when Basil Valentine allows his ire to get the better of him it is because of his indignation over the quacks who were abusing medicine and patients in his time, as they have ever since. There is a curious bit of aspersion on mere book learning in the passage that has a distinctly modern ring, and one feels the truth of Russell Lowell's expression that to read a classic, no matter how antique, is like reading a commentary on the morning paper, so up-to-date does genius ever remain:

> "And whensoever I shall have occasion to contend in the School with such a Doctor, who knows not how himself to prepare his own medicines, but commits that business to another, I am sure I shall obtain the Palm from him; For indeed that good man knows not what medicines he prescribes to the sick; whether the color of them be white, black, gray, or blew (*sic*), he cannot tell; nor doth this wretched man know whether the medicine he gives be dry or hot, cold or humid; but he only knows that he found it so written in his books, and then pretends to knowledge or as it were Possession by Prescription of a very long time; yet he desires to further information. Here again let it be lawful to exclaim, Good God, to what a state is the matter brought! what Goodness of Minde is in these men! what care do they take of the sick! Wo, wo to them! in the day of Judgement they will find the fruit of their Ignorance and Rashness, then they will see him whom they pierced, when they neglected their Neighbor, sought after money and nothing else; whereas were they cordial in their profession, they would spend Nights and

> Days in Labour that they might become more learned in their Art, whence more certain health would accrew to the sick with their estimation and greater glory to themselves. But since Labour is tedious to them they commit the matter to chance, and being secure of their Honour, and content with their Fame, they (like Brawlers) defend themselves with a certain garrulity, without any respect had to Confidence or Truth."

Perhaps one of the reasons why Valentine's book has been of such enduring interest is that it is written in an eminently human vein and out of a lively imagination. It is full of figures relating to many other things besides chemistry, which serve to show how deeply this investigating observer was attentive to all the problems of life around him. For instance, when he wants to describe the affinity that exists between many substances in chemistry, and which makes it impossible for them not to be attracted to one another, he takes a figure from the attractions that he sees exist among men and women. It is curious to find affinities discussed in our modern sense so long ago. There are some paragraphs with regard to the influence of the passion of love that one might think rather a quotation from an old-time sermon than from a great ground-breaking book in the science of chemistry.

> "Love leaves nothing entire or sound in man; it impedes his sleep, he cannot rest either day or night; it takes off his appetite that he hath no disposition either to meat or drink by reason of the continual torments of his heart and mind. It deprives him of all Providence, hence he neglects his affairs, vocation, and business. He minds neither study, labor, nor prayer;

> casts away all thoughts of anything but the body beloved; this is his study, this his most vain occupation. If to lovers the success be not answerable to their wish, or so soon and prosperously as they desire, how many melancholies henceforth arise, with griefs and sadness, with which they pine away and wax so lean as they have scarcely any flesh cleaving to the bones. Yea, at last they lose the life itself, as may be proved by many examples! for such men (which is an horrible thing to think of) slight and neglect all perils and detriments, both of the body and life, and of the soul and eternal salvation."

It is evident that human nature is not different in our sophisticated twentieth century from that which this observant old monk saw around him in the fifteenth. He continues:

> "How many testimonies of this violence which is in love, are daily found? for it not only inflames the younger sort, but it so far exaggerates some persons far gone in years as through the burning heat thereof, they are almost mad. Natural diseases are for the most part governed by the complexion of man and therefore invade some more fiercely, others more gently; but Love, without distinction of poor or rich, young or old, seizeth all, and having seized so blinds them as forgetting all rules of reason, they neither see nor hear any snare."

But then the old monk thinks that he has said enough about this rather foreign subject, and apologizes for his digression in another paragraph that should remove any lingering doubt there might be with regard to the genuineness of his monastic character. At the end of the passage he makes the application in a very few words. The personal element in his confession is so naïve and so simply straightforward that instead of seeming to be the result of conceit, which would surely have repelled the reader, it rather attracts and enhances his kindly feeling for its author. The paragraph would remind one in certain ways of that personal element that was to become more popular in literature after Montaigne in the next century made it rather the fashion.

> "But of these enough; for it becomes not a religious man to insist too long upon these cogitations, or to give place to such a flame in his heart. Hitherto (without boasting I speak it) I have throughout the whole course of my life kept myself safe and free from it, and I pray and invoke God to vouchsafe me his Grace that I may keep holy and inviolate the faith which I have sworn, and live contented with my spiritual spouse, the Holy Catholick Church. For no other reason have I alleged these than that I might express the love with which all tinctures ought to be moved towards metals, if ever they be admitted by them into true friendship, and by love, which permeates the inmost parts, be converted into a better state."

The application of the figure at the end of his long digression is characteristic of the period in which he wrote, as also to a considerable extent of the German literary methods of the time.

In this volume on the use of antimony there are in most of the editions certain biographical notes which have sometimes been accepted as authentic, but oftener rejected.

According to these, Basil Valentine was born in a town in Alsace, on the southern bank of the Rhine. As a consequence of this, there are several towns that have laid claim to being his birthplace. M. Jean Reynaud, the distinguished French philosophical writer of the first half of the nineteenth century, once said that Basil Valentine, like Ossian and Homer, had many towns claim him years after his death. He also suggested that, like those old poets, it was possible that the writings sometimes attributed to Basil Valentine were really the work not of one man, but of several individuals. There are, however, many objections to this theory, the most forcible of which is the internal evidence derived from the books themselves showing similarities of style and method of treating subjects too great for us to admit non-identity in the writers. M. Reynaud lived at a time when it was all the fashion to suggest that old works that had come down to us, like the Iliad and the Odyssey, and even such national epics as the Cid and the Arthur Legends and the Nibelungenlied were to be attributed to several writers rather than to one. We have passed that period of criticism, however, and have reverted to the idea of single authorship for these works, and the same conclusion has been generally come to with regard to the writings attributed to Basil Valentine.

Other biographic details contained in "The Triumphal Chariot of Antimony" are undoubtedly more correct. According to them Basil Valentine travelled in England

and Holland on missions for his order, and went through France and Spain on a pilgrimage to St. James of Compostella.

Besides this work, there is a number of other books of Basil Valentine's, printed during the first half of the sixteenth century, that are well known and copies of which may be found in most of the important libraries. The United States Surgeon General's Library at Washington contains not a few of the works on medical subjects, and the New York Academy of Medicine Library has some valuable editions of certain of his works. Some of his other well-known books, each of which is a good-sized octavo volume, bear the following descriptive titles (I give them in English, though as they are usually found, they are in Latin, sixteenth-century translations of the original German): "The World in Miniature: or, The Mystery of the World and of Human Medical Science," published at Mayburg, 1609; "The Chemical Apocalypse: or, The Manifestation of Artificial Chemical Compounds," published in Erfurt in 1624; "A Chemico-Philosophic Treatise Concerning Things Natural and Preternatural, Especially Relating to the Metals and the Minerals," published at Frankfurt in 1676; "Haliography: or, The Science of Salts: A Treatise on the Preparation, Use, and Chemical Properties of All the Mineral, Animal, and Vegetable Salts," published at Bologna in 1644; "The Twelve Keys of Philosophy," Leipsic, 1630. These are of interest to the chemist and physicist rather than to the physician, and it is as a Maker of Medicine that we are concerned with Valentine here.

The great attention aroused in Basil Valentine's work at the Renaissance period can be best realized from the number of manuscript copies and their wide distribution. His books were not all printed at one place, but, on the contrary, in different portions of Europe. The original edition of "The Triumphal Chariot of Antimony" was published in Leipsic in the early part of the sixteenth century. The first editions of the other books, however, appeared at places so distant from Leipsic as Amsterdam and Bologna, while various cities of Germany, as Erfurt and Frankfurt, claim the original editions of still other works. Many of the manuscript copies still exist in various libraries in Europe; and while there is no doubt that some unimportant additions to the supposed works of Basil Valentine have come from the attribution to him of scientific treatises of other German writers, the style and the method of the principal works mentioned is entirely too similar not to have been the fruit of a single mind and that possessed of a distinct investigating genius, setting it far above any of its contemporaries in scientific speculation and observation.

The most interesting feature of all of Basil Valentine's writings that are extant is the distinctive tendency to make his observations of special practical utility. His studies in antimony were made mainly with the idea of showing how that substance might be used in medicine. He did not neglect to point out other possible uses, however, and knew the secret of the employment of antimony in order to give sharpness and definition to the impression produced by metal types. It would seem as though he was the first scientist who discussed this subject, and there is even some question of whether printers and typefounders did not derive their ideas in this matter from our chemist.

Interested though he was in the transmutation of metals, he never failed to try to find and suggest some medicinal use for all of the substances that he investigated. His was no greedy search for gold and no cumulation of investigations with the idea of benefiting only himself. Mankind was always in his mind, and perhaps there is no better demonstration of his fulfilment of the character of the monk than this constant solicitude to benefit others by every bit of investigation that he carried out. For him, with medieval nobleness of spirit, "the first part of every work must be the invocation of God, and the last, though no less important than the first, must be the utility and fruit for mankind that can be derived from it."

The career of the last of the Makers of Medicine in the Middle Ages may be summed up briefly in a few sentences that show how thoroughly this old Benedictine was possessed of the spirit of modern science. He believed in observation as the most important source of medical knowledge. He valued clinical experience far above book information. He insisted on personal acquaintanceship on the part of the physician with the drugs he used, and thought nothing more unworthy of a practitioner of medicine,—indeed he sets it down as almost criminal—than to give remedies of whose composition he was not well aware and whose effect he did not thoroughly understand. He thought that nature was the most important aid to the physician, much more important than drugs, though he was the first to realize the significance of chemical affinities, and he seems to have understood rather well how individual often were the effects obtained from drugs. He was a patient student, a faithful observer, a writer who did not begrudge time and care to the composition of large books on medicine, yet withal he was no dry-as-dust scholar, but eminently human in his sympathies with ailing humanity, and a strenuous upholder of the dignity of the profession to which he belonged. Scarcely more can be said of anyone in the history of medicine, at least so far as good intentions go; though many accomplished more, none deserve more honor than the Thuringian monk whom we know as Basil Valentine.

There are many other of these old-time Makers of Medicine of whom nearly the same thing can be said. Basil Valentine is only one of a number of men who worked faithfully and did much both for medical science and professional life during the thousand years from the fall of Rome to the fall of Constantinople, when, according to what used to be commonly accepted opinion, men were not animated by the spirit of research and of fine incentive to do good to men that we are so likely to think of as belonging exclusively to more modern times. A man whom he greatly influenced, Paracelsus, took up the tradition of scientific investigation where Basil Valentine had left it. His work, though more successfully revolutionary, was not done in such a fine spirit of sympathy with humanity nor with that simplicity of life and purity of intention that characterized the old monk's work. Paracelsus' birth in the year of the discovery of America places him among the makers of the foundations of our modern medicine, and he will be treated of in a volume on "The Forefathers in Medicine."

APPENDIX I

ST. LUKE THE PHYSICIAN[32]

In the midst of what has been called the "higher criticism" of the Bible in recent times, one of the long accepted traditions that has been most strenuously assailed and, indeed, in the minds of many scholars, seemed, for a time at least, quite discredited, was that St. Luke the Evangelist, the author of the Third Gospel and the Acts of the Apostles, was a physician. Distinguished authorities in early Christian apologetics have declared that the pillars of primitive Christian history are the genuine Epistles of St.

Paul, the writings of St. Luke, and the history of Eusebius. It is quite easy to understand, then, that the attack upon the authenticity of the writings usually assigned to St. Luke, which in many minds seemed successful, has been considered of great importance. In the very recent time there has been a decided reaction in this matter. This has come, not so much from Roman Catholics, who have always clung to the traditional view, and whose great Biblical students have been foremost in the support of the previously accepted opinion, but from some of the most strenuous of the German higher critics, who now appreciate that destructive, so-called higher criticism went too far, and that the traditional view not only can be maintained, but is the only opinion that will adequately respond to all the new facts that have been found, and all the recently gathered information with regard to the relations of events in the olden time.

By far the most important contribution to the discussion in recent years came not long since from the pen of Professor Adolph Harnack, the professor of church history in the University of Berlin. Professor Harnack's name is usually cited as that of one of the most destructive of the higher critics. His recent book, however, "Luke the Physician,"[33] is an entire submission to the old-fashioned viewpoint that the writer of the Third Gospel and of the Acts of the Apostles was a Greek fellow-worker of St. Paul, who had been in company for years with Mark and Philip and James, and who had previously been a physician, and was evidently well versed in all the medical lore of that time. Harnack does not merely concede the old position. As might be expected, his rediscussion of the subject clinches the arguments for the traditional view, and makes it impossible ever to call it in question again. It is easy to understand how important are such admissions when we recall how much this traditional view has been assailed, and how those who have held it have been accused of old-fogyism and lack of scholarship, and unwarranted clinging to antiquated notions just because they thought they were of faith, and how, lacking in true scholarship, seriously hampering genuine investigation, such conservatism has been declared to be.

The question of Luke's having been a physician is an extremely valuable one, and no one in our time is better fitted by early training and long years of study to elucidate it than Professor Harnack. He began his excursions into historical writing years ago, as I understand, as an historian of early Christian medicine. Some of his works on medical conditions just before and after Christ are quoted confidently by the distinguished German medical historians. From this department he graduated into the field of the higher criticism. He is eminently in a position, therefore, to state the case with regard to St. Luke fully, and to indicate absolutely the conclusions that should be drawn from the premises of fact, writings, and traditions that we have. He does so in a very striking way. Perhaps no better example of his thoroughly lucid and eminently logical mode of argumentation is to be found than the paragraph in which he states the question. It might well be recommended as an example of terse forcefulness and logical sequence that deserves the emulation of all those who want to write on medical subjects. If we had more of these characteristic qualities of Harnack's style, our medical literature, so called, would not need to occupy so many pages of print as it does—yet would say more. Here it is:

> St. Luke, according to St. Paul, was a physician. When a physician writes a historical work it does not necessarily follow that his profession shows itself in his writing; yet it is only natural for one to look for traces of the author's medical profession in such a work. These traces may be of different kinds: 1, The whole character of the narrative may be determined by points of view, aims, and ideals which are more or less medical (disease and its treatment); 2, marked preference may be shown for stories concerning the healing of diseases, which stories may be given in great number and detail; 3, the language may be colored by the language of physicians (medical technical terms, metaphors of medical character, etc.). All these three groups of characteristic signs are found, as we shall see, in the historical work which bears the name of St. Luke. Here, however, it may be objected that the subject matter itself is responsible for these traits, so that their evidence is not decisive for the medical calling of the author. Jesus appeared as a great physician and healer. All the evangelists say this of Him; hence it is

> not surprising that one of them has set this phase of His ministry in the foreground, and has regarded it as the most important. Our evangelist need not therefore have been a physician, especially if he were a Greek, seeing that in those days Greeks with religious interests were disposed to regard religion mainly under the category of healing and salvation. This is true, yet such a combination of characteristic signs will compel us to believe that the author was a physician if, 4, the description of the particular cases of disease shows distinct traces of medical diagnosis and scientific knowledge; 5, if the language, even where questions of medicine or of healing are not touched upon, is colored by medical phraseology; and, 6, if in those passages where the author speaks as an eye-witness medical traits are especially and prominently apparent. These three kinds of tokens are also found in the historical work of our author. It is accordingly proved that it proceeds from the pen of a physician.

The importance of the concession that Luke was a physician should be properly appreciated. His whole gospel is written from that standpoint. For him the Saviour was the healer, the good physician who went about curing the ills of the body, while ministering to people's souls. He has more accounts of miracles of healing than any of the other Evangelists. He has taken certain of the stories of the other Evangelists who were eye-witnesses, and when they were told in naïve and popular language that obscured the real condition that was present, he has retold the story from the physician's standpoint, and thus the miracle becomes clearer than ever. In one case, where Mark has a slur on physicians, Luke eliminates it. In a number of cases the correction of Mark's popular language in the description of ailments is made in terms that could not have been used except by one thoroughly versed in the Greek medical terminology of the times. As a matter of fact, there seems to be no doubt now that Luke had been, before he became an Evangelist, a practising physician in Malta of considerable experience. His testimony, then, to the miracles is particularly valuable as almost a medical eye-witness.

In medical science, St. Luke's time was by no means barren of knowledge. The Alexandrian school of medicine had done some fine work in its time. It was the first university medical school in the world's history, and there dissection was first practised regularly and publicly for the sake of anatomy, and even the vivisection of criminals who were supplied by the Ptolemei for human physiology, was a part of the school curriculum. A number of important discoveries in brain anatomy are attributed to Herophilus, after whom the torcular herophili within the skull is named, and who invented the term calamus scriptorius for certain appearances in the fourth ventricle. His colleague, Erasistratus, the co-founder of this school at Alexandria, did work in pathological anatomy, and laid the foundation for serious study there. For three centuries there is some good worker, at or in connection with Alexandria, whose name is preserved for us in the history of medicine. Other Greek schools of medicine in the East, as, for instance, that of Pergamos, also did excellent work. Galen is the great representative of this school, and he came in the century after St. Luke. A physician educated in Greek medicine at that time, then, would be in an excellent position to judge critically of the miracles of healing of the Christ, and it would seem to have been providential that Luke was called for this purpose.

The evidence for his membership of our profession will doubtless be interesting to all physicians. Some of the distinctive passages in which Luke's familiarity with medical terms to such an extent that to express his meaning he found himself compelled to use them, will appeal at once to these, for whom such terms are part of everyday speech. The use of the word *hydropikos,* which is not to be met with anywhere else in the New Testament, nor in the non-medical Greek literature of that time, though the word is of frequent occurrence as a designation for a person suffering from dropsy (and always, as in Luke, the adjective for the substantive), in Hippocrates, Dioscorides, and Galen is a typical example.

Where such vague terms as paralyzed occur Luke does not use the familiar word, but the medical term that meant stricken with paralysis, indicating not any inability to use the limbs, but such a one as was due to a stroke of apoplexy. We who, as physicians, have heard of so many cures of paralysis from our friends, the Eddyites, are prone to ask, as the first question, what sort of a paralysis it was. Luke made inquiries from men who were eye-witnesses, and then has described the scene with such details as convinced him as a physician of the reality of the miracle, and his description was meant to carry conviction to the minds of others.

Occasionally St. Luke uses words which only a physician would be likely to know at all. That is to say, even a man reasonably familiar with medical terminology and medical literature would not be likely to know them unless he had been technically trained. One of these is the word *sphudron,* a word which is only medical, and is not to be found even in such large Greek lexicons of ordinary words as that of Passow. Sphudron is the anatomical term of the Græco-Alexandrian school for the condyles of the femur. Galen and other medical authors use it, and Luke, in giving the details of the story of the lame man cured, in the third chapter of the Acts, seventh verse, selects it because it exactly expresses the meaning he wished to convey. In this story there are a number of added medical details. These are all evidently arranged so as to give the full medical significance to the miracle. For instance, the man had been *lame from birth,* literally *from the womb of his mother.* At this time he was forty years of age, an age at which the spontaneous cure of such an ailment or, indeed, any cure of it, could scarcely be expected, if, during the preceding time, there had been no improvement.

In the story of the cure of Saul's blindness Luke says in the Acts that his blindness fell from him like scales. The figure is a typically medical one. The word for fall that is used is, as was pointed out by Hobart ("Medical Language of St. Luke," Dublin, 1882), exactly the term that is used for the falling of scales from the body. The term for scales is the specific designation of the particles that fall from the body during certain skin diseases or after certain of the infectious fevers, as in scarlet fever. Hippocrates and Galen have used it in many places. It is distinctively a medical word. In the story of the vision of St. Peter, told also in the Acts, the word *ecstasis,* from which we derive our word ecstasy, is used. This is the only word St. Luke uses for vision and he alone uses it. This term is of constant employment in a technical sense in the medical writers of St. Luke's time and before it. When the other evangelists talk of lame people they use the popular term. This might mean anything or nothing for a physician. Luke uses one of the terms that is employed by physicians when they wish to indicate that for some definite reason there is inability to walk.

In the story of the Good Samaritan there are some interesting details that indicate medical interest on the part of the writer. It is Luke's characteristic story and a typical medical instance. He employs certain words in it that are used only by medical writers. The use of oil and wine in the treatment of the wounds of the stranger traveller was at one time said to indicate that it could not have been a physician who wrote the story, since the ancients used oil for external applications in such cases but not wine. More careful search of the old masters of medicine, however, has shown that they used oil and wine not only internally but externally. Hippocrates, for instance, has a number of recommendations of this combination for wounds. It is rather interesting to realize this, and especially the wine in addition to the oil, because wine contains enough alcohol to be rather satisfactorily antiseptic. There seems no doubt that wounds that had been bathed in wine and then had oil poured over them would be likely to do better than those which were treated in other ways. The wine would cleanse and at least inhibit bacterial growth. The subsequent covering with oil would serve to protect the wound to some degree from external contamination.

Sometimes there is an application of medical terms to something extraneous from medicine that makes the phrase employed quite amusing. For instance, when Luke wants to explain how they strengthened the vessel in which they were to sail he describes the process by the term which was used in medical Greek to mean the splinting of a part or at least the binding of it up in such a way as to enable it to be used. The word was quite a puzzle to the commentators until it was pointed out that it was the familiar medical term, and then it was easy to understand. Occasionally this use of a medical term gives a strikingly accurate significance to Luke's diction. For instance, where other evangelists talk of the Lord looking at a patient or turning to them, Luke uses the expression that was technically employed for a physician's examination of his patient, as if the Lord carefully looked over the ailing people to see their physical needs, and then proceeded to cure them. Manifestly in Luke's mind the most interesting phase of the Lord's life was His exhibition of curative powers, and the Saviour was for him the divine healer, the God physician of bodies as well as of souls.

There are many little incidents which he relates that emphasize this. For instance, where St. Mark talks about the healing of the man with a withered hand, St. Luke adds the characteristic medical note that it was the right hand. When he tells of the cutting off of the ear of the servant of the high priest in the Garden of Olives St. Luke takes the story from St. Mark, but adds the information that would appeal to a physician that it was the right ear. Moreover, though all four evangelists record the cutting off of the ear, only St. Luke adds the information that the Lord healed it again. It is as if he were defending the kindly feelings of the Divine Physician and as if it would have been inexcusable had He not exerted His miraculous powers of healing on this occasion. It is St. Luke, too, who has constantly distinguished between natural illnesses and cases of possession. This careful distinction alone would point to the author of the third gospel and the Acts as surely a physician. As it is it confirms beyond all doubt the claim that the writer of these portions of the New Testament was a physician thoroughly familiar with all the medical writings of the time and probably a physician who had practised for a long time.

Certain miracles of healing are related only by St. Luke as if he realized better than any of the other evangelists the evidential value that such instances would have for future generations as to the divinity of the personage who worked them. The beautiful story of the raising from death of the son of the widow of Nain is probably one of the oftenest quoted passages from St. Luke. It is a charming bit of literature. While it suggests the writer physician it makes one almost sure that the other tradition according to which St. Luke was also a painter must be true. The scene is as picturesque as it can be. The Lord and His Apostles and the multitudes coming to the gate of the little city just as in the evening sun the funeral cortège with the widow burying her only son came out of it. The approach of the Lord to the weeping mother, His command to the dead son to arise, and the simple words, "and he gave him back to his mother," constitute as charming a scene as a painter ever tried to visualize. Besides this, Luke alone has the story of the man suffering with dropsy and the woman suffering from weakness. The intensely picturesque quality of many of these scenes that he describes so vividly would indeed seem to place beyond all doubt the old tradition that he was an artist as well as a physician.

It is interesting to realize that it is to Luke alone that we owe the account of the well-known message sent by Christ Himself to John the Baptist when John sent his disciples to inquire as to His mission. After describing His ministry He said: "Go and relate to John what you have heard and seen: the blind see, the lame walk, the deaf hear, the lepers are made clean, the dead rise again, to the poor the Gospel is preached." To no one more than to a physician would that description of His mission appeal as surely divine.

To those who care to follow the subject still further, and above all, to read opinions given before the reversal of the verdict of the higher criticism on the Lucan writings, indeed before ever that trial was brought, there is much in "Horæ Lucanæ—A Biography of St. Luke," by Henry Samuel Baynes (Longmans, 1870), that will surely be of interest. He has some interesting quotations which show how thoroughly previous centuries realized all the force of modern arguments. For instance, the following paragraph from Dr. Nathaniel Robinson, a Scotch physician of the eighteenth century, will illustrate this. Dr. Robinson said:

> It is manifest from his Gospel, that Luke was both an acute observer, and had even given professional attention to all our Saviour's miracles of healing. Originally, among the Egyptians, divinity and physic were united in the same order of men, so that the priest had the care of souls, and was also the physician. It was much the same under the Jewish economy. But after physic came to be studied by the Greeks, they separated the two

> professions. That a physician should write the history of our Saviour's life was appropriate, as there were divers mysterious things to be noticed, concerning which his education enabled him to form a becoming judgment.

It is even interesting to realize that St. Luke's tendency to use medical terms has been of definite value in determining the question whether both the third gospel and the Acts of the Apostles are by the same man. They have been attributed to St. Luke traditionally, but in the higher criticism some doubt has been thrown on this and an elaborate hypothesis of dual authorship set up. It has been asserted that it is very improbable on extrinsic grounds that they were both written by one hand and certain intrinsic evidence, changes in the mode of narration, especially the use of the first personal pronoun in the plural in certain passages, has been pointed to as making against single authorship. This tendency to deny old-time traditions of authorship with regard to many classical writings was a marked characteristic of the early part of the nineteenth century, but the close of the century saw practically all of these denials discredited. The nineteenth century ushered in studies of Homer, with the separatist school perfectly confident in their assertion that the Iliad and the Odyssey were not by the same person, and even that the Iliad itself was the work of several hands.

At the beginning of the twentieth century we are quite as sure that both the Iliad and Odyssey were written by the same person and that the separatists were hurried into a contrary decision not a little by the feeling of the sensation that such a contradiction of previously accepted ideas would create. This is a determining factor in many a supposed novel discovery, that it is hard always to discount sufficiently. A thing may be right even though it is old, and most new discoveries, it must not be forgotten, that is, most of those announced with a great blare of trumpets, do not maintain themselves. The simple argument that the separatists would have to find another poet equal to Homer to write the other poem has done more than anything else to bring their opinion into disrepute. It is much easier to explain certain discrepancies, differences of style, and of treatment of subjects, as well as other minor variants, than to supply another great poet. Most of the works of our older literatures have gone through a similar trial during the over-hasty superficially critical nineteenth century. The Nibelungenlied has been attributed to two or three writers instead of one. The Cid, the national epic of Spain, and the Arthur Legends, the first British epic, have been at least supposed to be amenable to the same sort of criticism. In every case, scholars have gone back to the older traditional view of a single author. The phases of literary and historic criticism with regard to Luke's writings are, then, only a repetition of what all our great national classics have gone through from supercilious scholarship during the past hundred years.

It is not surprising, then, that there should be dual or even triple ascriptions of authorship for various portions of the Scriptures, and Luke's writings have on this score suffered as much or more even than others, with the possible exception of Moses. It is now definitely settled, however, that the similarities of style between the Acts and the third gospel are too great for them to have come from two different minds. This is especially true, as pointed out by Harnack, in all that regards the use of medical terms. The writer of the Acts and the writer of the third gospel knew Greek from the standpoint of the physician of that time. Each used terms that we find nowhere else in Greek literature except among medical writers. What is thus true for one critical attack on Luke's reputation is also true in another phase of recent higher criticism. It has been said that certain portions of the Acts which are called the "we" portions because the narration changes in them from the third to the first person were to be attributed to another writer than the one who wrote the narrative portions. Here, once more, the test of the medical words employed has decided the case for Luke's sole authorship. It is evidently an excellent thing to be able to use medical terms properly if one wants to be recognized with certainty later on in history for just what one's business was. It has certainly saved the situation for St. Luke, though there may be some doubt as to the real force of objections thus easily overthrown.

It is rather interesting to realize that many scholars of the present generation had allowed themselves to be led away by the German higher criticism from the old tradition with regard to Luke as a physician and now will doubtless be led back to former views by the leader of German biblical critics. It shows how much more distant things may influence certain people than those nearer home—how the hills are green far away. Harnack confesses that the best book ever written on the subject of Luke as a physician, the one that has proved of most value to him, and that he still recommends everyone to read, was originally written in English. It is Hobart's "Medical Language of St. Luke,"[34] written more than a quarter of a century before Harnack. The Germans generally had rather despised what the English were doing in the matter of biblical criticism, and above all in philology. Yet now the acknowledged coryphæus of them all, Harnack, not only admits the superiority of an old-time English book, but confesses that it is the best statement of the subject up to the present time, including his own. He constantly quotes from it, and it is evident that it has been the foundation of all of his arguments. It is not the first time that men have fetched from afar what they might have got just as well or better at home.

Harnack has made complete the demonstration,then, that the third gospel and the Acts were written by St. Luke, who had been a practising physician. In spite of this, however, he finds many objections to the Luke narratives and considers that they add very little that is valuable to the contemporary evidence that we have with regard to Christ. He impairs with one hand the value of what he has so lavishly yielded with the other. He finds inconsistencies and discrepancies in the narrative that for him destroy their value as testimony. A lawyer would probably say that this is that very human element in the writings which demonstrates their authenticity and adds to their value as evidence, because it shows clearly the lack of any attempt to do anything more than tell a direct story as it had come to the narrator. No special effort was made to avoid critical objections founded on details. It was the general impression that was looked for.

Sir William Ramsay, in his "Luke the Physician and Other Studies in the History of Religion" (New York: Armstrong and Sons, 1908), has answered Harnack from the side of the professional critic with much force. He appreciates thoroughly the value of Professor Harnack's book, and above all the reactionary tendency away from nihilistic so-called higher criticism which characterized so much of German writing on biblical themes in the nineteenth century. He says (p. 7): "This [book of Harnack's] alone carries Lukan criticism a long step forwards, and sets it on a new and higher plane. Never has the unity and character of the book been demonstrated so convincingly and conclusively. The step is made and the plane is reached by the method which is practised in other departments of literary criticism, viz., by dispassionate investigation of the work and by discarding fashionable *a priori* theories."

The distinguished English traveller and writer on biblical subjects points out, however, that in detail many of

Harnack's objections to the Lukan narratives are due to insufficient consideration of the circumstances in which they were written and the comparative significance of the details criticised. He says, "Harnack lays much stress on the fact that inconsistencies and inexactnesses occur all through Acts. Some of these are undeniable; and I have argued that they are to be regarded in the same light as similar phenomena in the poem of Lucretius and in other ancient classical writers, viz., as proofs that the work never received the final form which Luke intended to give it, but was still incomplete when he died. The evident need for a third book to complete the work, together with those blemishes in expression, form the proof."

Ramsay's placing of Harnack's writing in general is interesting in this connection. (P. 8) "Professor Harnack stands on the border between the nineteenth and twentieth century. His book shows that he is to a certain degree sensitive of and obedient to the new spirit; but he is only partially so. The nineteenth century critical method was false, and is already antiquated....

"The first century could find nothing real and true that was not accompanied by the marvellous and the 'supernatural.' The nineteenth century could find nothing real and true that was. Which view was right and which was wrong? Was either complete? Of these two questions, the second alone is profitable at the present. Both views were right—in a certain way of contemplating; both views were wrong—in a certain way. Neither was complete. At present, as we are struggling to throw off the fetters which impeded thought in the nineteenth century, it is most important to free ourselves from its prejudices and narrowness."

He adds (pp. 26 and 27): "There are clear signs of the unfinished state in which this chapter was left by Luke; but some of the German scholar's criticisms show that he has not a right idea of the simplicity of life and equipment that evidently characterized the jailer's house and the prison. The details which he blames as inexact and inconsistent are sometimes most instructive about the circumstances of this provincial town and Roman colonia.

"But it is never safe to lay much stress on small points of inexactness or inconsistency in any author. One finds such faults even in the works of modern scholarship if one examines them in the microscopic fashion in which Luke is studied here. I think I can find them in the author [Harnack] himself. His point of view sometimes varies in a puzzling way."

As a matter of fact, Harnack, as pointed out by Ramsay, was evidently working himself more and more out of the old conclusion as to the lack of authenticity of the Lucan writings into an opinion ever more and more favorable to Luke. For instance, in a notice of his own book, published in the *Theologische Literaturzeitung,* "he speaks far more favorably about the trustworthiness and credibility of

Luke, as being generally in a position to acquire and transmit reliable information, and as having proved himself able to take advantage of his position. Harnack was gradually working his way to a new plane of thought. His later opinion is more favorable."

Ramsay also points out that Professor Giffert, one of our American biblical critics, had felt compelled by the geographical and historical evidence to abandon in part the older unfavorable criticism of Luke and to admit that the Acts is more trustworthy than previous critics allowed. Above all, "he saw that it was a living piece of literature written by one author." In a word, Luke is being vindicated in every regard.

Some of the supposed inaccuracies of Luke vanish when careful investigation is made. Some of his natural history details, for instance, have been impugned and the story of the viper that "fastened" itself upon St. Paul in Malta has been cited as an example of a story that would not have been told in that way by a man who knew medicine and the related sciences in Luke's time. Because the passage illustrates a number of phases of the discussion with regard to Luke's language I make a rather long quotation from Ramsay:

> Take as a specimen with which to finish off this paper the passage Acts xxviii, 9 *et seq.*, which is very fully discussed by Harnack twice. He argues that the true meaning of the passage was not understood until medical

language was compared, when it was shown that the Greek word by which the act of the viper to Paul's hand is described, implies "bit" and not merely "fastened upon." But it is a well-assured fact that the viper, a poisonous snake, only strikes, fixes the poison fangs on the flesh for a moment, and withdraws its head instantly. Its action could never be what is attributed by Luke the eye witness to this Maltese viper; that it hung from Paul's hand and was shaken off into the fire by him. On the other hand, constrictors, which have no poison fangs, cling in the way described, but as a rule do not bite. Are we, then, to understand in spite of the medical style and the authority of Professor Blass (who translates "momordit" in his edition), that the viper fastened upon the apostle's hand? Then, the very name viper is a difficulty. Was Luke mistaken about the kind of snake which he saw? A trained medical man in ancient times was usually a good authority about serpents, to which great respect was paid in ancient medicine and custom.

Mere verbal study is here utterly at fault. We can make no progress without turning to the realities and facts of Maltese natural history. A correspondent obligingly informed me some years ago that Mr. Bryan Hook, of Farnham, Surrey (who, my correspondent assures me, is a thoroughly good naturalist), had found in Malta a small snake, *Coronella austriaca,* which is rare in England, but common in many parts of Europe. It is a constrictor, without poison fangs, which would cling to the hand or arm as Luke describes. It is similar in size to the viper, and so like in markings and general appearance that Mr. Hook, when he caught his specimen, thought he was killing a viper.

My friend, Prof. J. W. H. Trail, of Aberdeen, whom I consulted, replied that *Coronella lævis* or *austriaca,* is known in Sicily and the adjoining islands; but he can find no evidence of its existence in Malta. It is known to be rather irritable, and to fix its small teeth so firmly into the human skin as to need a little force to pull it off, though the teeth are too short to do any real injury to the skin. Coronella is at a glance very much like a viper; and in the flames it would not be closely examined. While it is not reported as found in Malta except by Mr. Hook, two species are known there belonging to the same family and having similar habits (*leopardinus* and *zamenis* (or *coluber*) *gemonensis*). The coloring of *Coronella leopardinus* would be the most likely to suggest a viper.

The observations justify Luke entirely. We have here a snake so closely resembling a viper as to be taken for one by a good naturalist until he had caught and examined a specimen. It clings, and yet it also bites without doing harm. That the Maltese rustics should mistake this harmless snake for a venomous one is not strange. Many uneducated people have the idea that all snakes are poisonous in varying degrees, just as the vulgar often firmly believe that toads are poisonous. Every detail as related by Luke is natural, and in accordance with the facts of the country.

> In a word, then, the whole question as to Luke's authority as a writer, as an eye-witness of many things, and as the relator of many others with regard to which he had obtained the testimony of eye-witnesses is fully vindicated. Twenty years ago many scholars were prone to doubt this whole question. Ten years ago most of them were convinced that the Luke traditions were not justified by recent investigation. Now we have come back once more to the complete acceptance of the old traditions.

Perhaps the most unfortunate characteristic of much nineteenth-century criticism in all departments, even those strictly scientific, was the marked tendency to reject previous opinions for new ones. Somehow men felt themselves so far ahead of old-time writers and thinkers that they concluded they must hold opinions different from their ancestors. In nearly every case the new ideas that they evolved by supposedly newer methods are not standing the test of time and further study. There had been a continuous belief in men's minds, having its basis very probably on a passage in one of St. Peter's Epistles, that the earth would dissolve by fire. This was openly contradicted all during the nineteenth century and the time when the earth would freeze up definitely calculated by our mathematicians.Now after having studied radioactivity and learned from the physicist that the earth is heating up and will eventually get too hot for life, we calmly go back to the old Petrine declaration. Some of the most distinguished of the German biologists of the present day, such men as Driesch and others, calmly tell us that the edifice erected by Darwin will have to come down because of newly discovered evidence, and indeed some of them go so far as to declare that Darwinism was a crude hypothesis very superficial in its philosophical aspects and therefore acceptable to a great many people who, because it was easy to understand and was very different from what our fathers had believed, hastened to accept it. Nothing shows the necessity for being conservative in the matter of new views in science or ethics or religion more than the curious transition state in which we are with regard to many opinions at the present time, with a distinct tendency toward reaction to older views that a few years ago were thought quite untenable. We are rather proud of the advance that we are supposed to be making along many lines in science and scholarship, and yet over and over again, after years of work, we prove to have been following a wrong lead and must come back to where we started. This has been the way of man from the beginning and doubtless will continue. The present generation are having this curious regression that follows supposed progress strongly emphasized for them.

APPENDIX II

SCIENCE AT THE MEDIEVAL UNIVERSITIES[35]

With the growth of interest in science and in nature study in our own day, one of the expressions that is probably oftenest heard is surprise that the men of preceding generations and especially university men did not occupy themselves more with the world around them and with the phenomena that are so tempting to curiosity. Science is usually supposed to be comparatively new and nature study only a few generations old. Men are supposed to have been so much interested in book knowledge and in speculations and theories of many kinds, that they neglected the realities of life around them while spinning fine webs of theory. Previous generations, of course, have indulged in theory, but then our own generation is not entirely free from that amusing occupation. Nothing could well be less true, however, than that the men of preceding generations were not interested in science even in the sense of physical science, or that nature study is new, or that men were not curious and did not try to find out all they could about the phenomena of the world around them.

The medieval universities and the school-men who taught in them have been particularly blamed for their failure to occupy themselves with realities instead of with speculation. We are coming to recognize their wonderful zeal for education, the large numbers of students they attracted, the enthusiasm of their students, since they made so many handwritten copies of the books of their masters, the devotion of the teachers themselves, who wrote at much greater length than do our professors even now and on the most abstruse subjects, so that it is all the more surprising to think they should have neglected science. The thought of our generation in the matter, however, is founded entirely on an assumption. Those who know anything about the writers of the Middle Ages at first hand are not likely to think of them as neglectful of science even in our sense of the term. Those who know them at second hand are, however, very sure in the matter.

The assumption is due to the neglect of history that came in the seventeenth and eighteenth centuries. We have many other similar assumptions because of the neglect of many phases of mental development and applied science at this time. For instance, most of us are very proud of our modern hospital development and think of this as a great humanitarian evolution of applied medical science. We are very likely to think that this is the first time in the world's history that the building of hospitals has been brought to such a climax of development, and that the houses for the ailing in the olden time were mere refuges, prone to become death traps and at most makeshifts for the solution of the problem of the care of the ailing poor. This is true for the hospitals of the seventeenth and eighteenth centuries, but it is not true at all for the hospitals of the thirteenth and fourteenth and fifteenth centuries. Miss Nutting and Miss Dock in their "History of Nursing"[36] have called attention to the fact that the lowest period in hospital development is during the eighteenth and early nineteenth centuries. Hospitals were little better than prisons, they had narrow windows, were ill provided with light and air and hygienic arrangements, and in general were all that we should imagine old-time hospitals to be. The hospitals of the earlier time, however, had fine high ceilings, large windows, abundant light and air, excellent arrangements for the privacy of patients, and in general were as worthy of the architects of the earlier times as the municipal buildings, the cathedrals, the castles, the university buildings, and every other form of construction that the late medieval centuries devoted themselves to.

The trouble with those who assume that there was no study of science and practically no attention to nature study in the Middle Ages is that they know nothing at all at first hand about the works of the men who wrote in the medieval period. They have accepted declarations with regard to the absolute dependence of the scholastics on authority, their almost divine worship of Aristotle, their utter readiness to accept authoritative assertions provided they came with the stamp of a mighty name, and then their complete lack of attention to observation and above all to experiment. Nothing could well be more ridiculous than this ignorant assumption of knowledge with regard to the great teachers at the medieval universities. Just as soon as there is definite knowledge of what these great teachers wrote and taught, not only does the previous mood of blame for them for not paying much more attention to science and nature at once disappear, but it gives place to the heartiest admiration for the work of these great thinkers. It is easy to appreciate, then, what Professor Saintsbury said in a recent volume on the thirteenth century:

> And there have even been in these latter days some graceless ones who have asked whether the science of the nineteenth century after an equal interval will be of any more positive value—whether it will not have even less comparative interest than that which appertains to the scholasticism of the thirteenth.

Three men were the great teachers in the medieval universities at their prime. They have been read and studied with interest ever since. They wrote huge tomes, but men have pored over them in every generation. They were Albertus Magnus, the teacher of the other two, Thomas Aquinas and Roger Bacon. All three of them were together at the University of Paris shortly after the middle of the thirteenth century. Anyone who wants to know anything about the attitude of mind of the medieval universities, their professors and students, and of all the intellectual world of the time towards science and observation and experiment, should read the books of these men. Any other mode of getting at any knowledge of the real significance of the science of this time is mere pretence. These constitute the documents behind any scientific history of the development of science at this time. It is extremely interesting to see the attitude of these men with regard to authority. In Albert's tenth book (of his "Summa"), in which he catalogues and describes all the trees, plants, and herbs known in his time, he observes: "All that is here set down is the result of our own experience, or has been borrowed from authors whom we know to have written what their personal experience has confirmed; for in these matters experience alone can be of certainty." In his impressive Latin phrase "*experimentum solum certificat in talibus*." With regard to the study of nature in general he was quite as emphatic. He was a theologian as well as a scientist, yet in his treatise on "The Heavens and the Earth" he declared that "in studying nature we have not to inquire how God the Creator may, as He freely wills, use His creatures to work miracles and thereby show forth His power. We have rather to inquire what nature with its immanent causes can naturally bring to pass."[37]

Just as striking quotations on this subject might be made from Roger Bacon. Indeed, Bacon was quite impatient with the scholars around him who talked over-much, did not observe enough, depended to excess on authority, and in general did as mediocre scholars always do, made much fuss on second-hand information—plus some filmy speculations of their own. Friar Bacon, however, had one great pupil whose work he thoroughly appreciated because it exhibited the opposite qualities. This was Petrus —we have come to know him as Peregrinus—whose observations on magnetism have excited so much attention in recent years with the republications of his epistle on the subject. It is really a monograph on magnetism written in the thirteenth century. Roger Bacon's opinion of it and of its author furnishes us the best possible index of his attitude of mind towards observation and experiment in science.

> I know of only one person who deserves praise for his work in experimental philosophy for he does not care for the discourses of men and their wordy warfare, but quietly and diligently pursues the works of wisdom. Therefore what others grope after blindly, as bats in the evening twilight, this man contemplates in their brilliancy *because he is a master of experiment*. Hence, he knows all of natural science whether pertaining to medicine and alchemy, or to matters celestial or terrestrial. He has worked diligently in the smelting of ores as also in the working of minerals; he is thoroughly acquainted with all sorts of arms and implements used in military service and in hunting, besides which he is skilled in agriculture and in the measurement of lands. It is impossible to write a useful or correct treatise in experimental philosophy without mentioning this man's name.

> Moreover, he pursues knowledge for its own sake; for if he wished to obtain royal favor, he could easily find sovereigns who would honor and enrich him.

Similar expressions might readily be quoted from Thomas Aquinas, but his works are so easy to secure and his whole attitude of mind so well known, that it scarcely seems worth while taking space to do so. Aquinas is still studied very faithfully in many universities, and within the last few years one of his great text-books of philosophy has been replaced in the curriculum of Oxford University, in which it occupied a prominent position in the long ago, as a work that may be offered for examination in the department of philosophy. It is with regard to him particularly that there has been the greatest revulsion of feeling in recent years and a recognition of the fact that here was a great thinker familiar with all that was known in the physical sciences, and who had this knowledge constantly in his mind when he drew his conclusions with regard to philosophical and theological questions.

It used to be the fashion to make little of the medieval scholars for the high estimation in which they held Aristotle. Occasionally even yet one hears narrowly educated men, I am sorry to say much more frequently scientific specialists than others, talk deprecatingly of this ardent devotion to Aristotle. No one who knows anything about Aristotle ever indulges in such an exhibition of ignorance of the realities of the history of philosophy and science. To know Aristotle well is to think of him as probably possessed of the greatest human mind that ever existed. We do not need to go back to the Middle Ages to be confirmed in that opinion. Modern scientists who know their science well, but who also know Aristotle well, and who are ardent worshippers at his shrine, are not hard to find. Romanes, the great English biologist of the end of the nineteenth century, said: "It appears to me that there can be no question that Aristotle stands forth not only as the greatest figure in antiquity but as the greatest intellect that has ever appeared upon this earth."

Before Romanes, George H. Lewes, in his interesting monograph in the history of thought, "Aristotle, a Chapter in the History of Science," is quite as complimentary to the great Greek thinker. We may say that Lewes was by no means partial to Aristotle. Anything but inclined to accept authority as of value in philosophy, he had been rendered impatient by the fact that so much of the history of philosophy was dominated by Aristotle, and it was only that the panegyric was forced from him by careful study of all that the Stagirite wrote that he said: "History gazed on him with wonder. His intellect was piercing and comprehensive; his attainments surpassed those of every philosopher; his influence has been excelled only by the founders of religion ... his vast and active intelligence for twenty centuries held the world in awe."

Professor Osborn, whose scholarly study of the theory of evolution down the ages "From the Greeks to Darwin" rather startled the world of science by showing not only how old was a theory of evolution, but how frequently it had been stated and how many of them anticipated phases of our own thought in the matter, pays a high compliment to the great Greek scientist. He says: "Aristotle clearly states and rejects a theory of the origin of adaptive structures in animals altogether similar to that of Darwin." He then quotes certain passages from Aristotle's "Physics," and says: "These passages seem to contain absolute evidence that Aristotle had substantially the modern conception of the evolution of life, from a primordial, soft mass of living matter to the most perfect forms, and that even in these he believed that evolution was incomplete for they were progressing to higher forms."

Modern French scientists are particularly laudatory in their estimation of Aristotle. The group of biologists, Buffon, Cuvier, St. Hilaire, and others who called world attention to French science and its attainments about a century ago, are all of them on record in highest praise of Aristotle. Cuvier said: "I cannot read his work without being ravished with astonishment. It is impossible to conceive how a single man was able to collect and compare the multitude of facts implied in the rules and aphorisms contained in this book."

It is possible, however, to get opinions ardently laudatory of Aristotle from the serious students of any nation, provided only they know their Aristotle. Sir William Hamilton, the Scotch philosopher, said:

"Aristotle's seal is upon all the sciences, his speculations have determined those of all subsequent thinkers." Hegel, the German philosophic writer, is not less outspoken in his praise: "Aristotle penetrated the whole universe of things and subjected them to intelligence." Kant, who is often said to have influenced our modern thinking more than any other in recent generations, has his compliment for Aristotle. It relates particularly to that branch of philosophy with which Kant had most occupied himself. The Koenigsberg philosopher said: "Logic since Aristotle, like Geometry since Euclid, is a finished science."

I do not want to tire you or I could quote many other authorities who proclaim Aristotle the genius of the race. They would include poets like Dante and Goethe, scholars like Cicero and Anthon, literary men like Lessing and Reich and many others. The scholars of the Middle Ages, far from condemnation for their devotion to Aristotle, deserve the highest praise for it. If they had done nothing else but appreciate Aristotle as our greatest modern scholars have done, that of itself would proclaim their profound scholarship.

The medieval writers are often said to have been uncritical in their judgment, but in their lofty estimation of Aristotle they displayed the finest possible critical judgment. On the contrary, the generations who made much of the opportunity to minimize medieval scholarship because of its worship at the shrine of Aristotle, must themselves fall under the suspicion at least of either not knowing Aristotle or of not thinking deeply about the subjects with regard to which he wrote. For in all the world's history the rule has been that whenever men have thought deeply about a subject and know what Aristotle has written with regard to that subject, they have the liveliest admiration for the great Greek thinker. This is true for philosophy, logic, metaphysics, politics, ethics, dramatics, but it is also quite as true for physical science. He lacked our knowledge, though not nearly to the degree that is usually thought, and he had a marvellous accumulation of information, but he had a breadth of view and a thoroughness of appreciation with a power of penetration that make his opinions worth while knowing even on scientific subjects in our enlightened age.

As for the supposed swearing by Aristotle, in the sense of literally accepting his opinions without daring to examine them critically, which is so constantly asserted to have been the habit of the medieval scholars and teachers, it is extremely difficult in the light of the expressions which we have from them, to understand how this false impression arose. Aristotle they thoroughly respected. They constantly referred to his works, but so has every thinking generation ever since. Whenever he had made a declaration they would not accept the contradiction of it without a good reason, but whenever they had good reasons, Aristotle's opinion was at once rejected without compunction. Albertus Magnus, for instance, said:

"Whoever believes that Aristotle was a God must also believe that he never erred,but if we believe that Aristotle was a man, then doubtless he was liable to err just as we are." A number of direct contradictions of Aristotle we have from Albert. A well-known one is that with regard to Aristotle's assertion that lunar rainbows appeared only twice in fifty years. Albert declared that he himself had seen two in a single year.

Indeed, it seems very clear that the whole trend of thought among the great teachers of the time was away from the acceptance of scientific conclusions on authority unless there was good evidence for them available. They were quite as impatient as the scientists of our time with the constant putting forward of Aristotle as if that settled a scientific question. Roger Bacon wanted the Pope to forbid the study of Aristotle because his works were leading men astray from the study of science, his authority being looked upon as so great that men did not think for themselves but accepted his assertions. Smaller men are always prone to do this, and indeed it constitutes one of the difficulties in the way of advance in scientific knowledge at all times, as Roger Bacon himself pointed out.

These are the sort of expressions that are to be expected from Friar Bacon from what we know of other parts of his work. His "Opus Tertium" was written at the request of Pope Clement IV, because the Pope had heard many interesting accounts of what the great thirteenth-century teacher and experimenter was doing at the University of Oxford, and wished to learn for himself the details of his work. Bacon starts out with the principle that there are four grounds of human ignorance. These are, "first, trust in inadequate authority; second, that force of custom which leads men to accept without properly questioning what has been accepted before their time; third, the placing of confidence in the assertions of the inexperienced; and fourth, the hiding of one's own ignorance behind the parade of superficial knowledge, so that we are afraid to say I do not know." Professor Henry Morley, a careful student of Bacon's writings, said with regard to these expressions of Bacon:

> No part of that ground has yet been cut away from beneath the feet of students, although six centuries have passed. We still make sheep-walks of second, third and fourth, and fiftieth hand references to authority; still we are the slaves of habit, still we are found following too frequently the untaught crowd, still we flinch from the righteous and wholesome phrase "I do not know" and acquiesce actively in the opinion of others that we know what we appear to know.

In his "Opus Majus" Bacon had previously given abundant evidence of his respect for the experimental method. There is a section of this work which bears the title "Scientia Experimentalis." In this Bacon affirms that "without experiment nothing can be adequately known. An argument may prove the correctness of a theory, but does not give the certitude necessary to remove all doubt, nor will the mind repose in the clear view of truth unless it finds its way by means of experiment." To this he later added in his "Opus Tertium": "The strongest argument proves nothing so long as the conclusions are not verified by experience. Experimental science is the queen of sciences, and the goal of all speculation."

It is no wonder that Dr. Whewell, in his "History of the Inductive Sciences," should have been unstinted in his praise of Roger Bacon's work and writings. In a well-known passage he says of the "Opus Majus":

> Roger Bacon's "Opus Majus" is the encyclopedia and "Novum Organon" of the thirteenth century, a work equally wonderful with regard to its wonderful scheme and to the special treatises by which the outlines of the plans are filled up. The professed object of the work is to urge the necessity of a reform in the mode of philosophizing, to set forth the reasons why knowledge had not made greater progress, to draw back attention to the sources of knowl edge which had been unwisely neglected, to discover other sources which were yet almost untouched, and to animate men in the undertaking of a prospect of the vast advantages which it offered. In the development of this plan all the leading portions of science are expanded in the most complete shape which they had at that time assumed; and improvements of a very wide and striking kind are proposed in some of the principal branches of study. Even if the work had no leading purposes it would have been highly valuable as a treasure of the most solid knowledge and soundest speculations of the

> time; even if it had contained no such details it would have been a work most remarkable for its general views and scope.

As a matter of fact the universities of the Middle Ages, far from neglecting science, were really scientific universities. Because the universities of the early nineteenth century occupied themselves almost exclusively with languages and especially formed students' minds by means of classical studies, men in our time seem to be prone to think that such linguistic studies formed the main portion of the curriculum of the universities in all the old times and particularly in the Middle Ages. The study of the classic languages, however, came into university life only after the Renaissance. Before that the undergraduates of the universities had occupied themselves almost entirely with science. It was quite as much trouble to introduce linguistic studies into the old universities in the Renaissance time to replace science, as it was to secure room for science by pushing out the classics in the modern time. Indeed the two revolutions in education are strikingly similar when studied in detail. Men who had been brought up on science before the Renaissance were quite sure that that formed the best possible means of developing the mind. In the early nineteenth century men who had been formed on the classics were quite as sure that science could not replace them with any success. There is no pretence that this view of the medieval universities is a new idea in the history of education. Those who have known the old universities at first hand by the study of the actual books of their professors and by familiarity with their courses of study, have not been inclined to make the mistake of thinking that the medieval university neglected science. Professor Huxley in his "Inaugural Address as Rector of Aberdeen University" some thirty years ago stated very definitely his recognition of medieval devotion to science. His words are well worth remembering by all those who are accustomed to think of our time as the first in which the study of science was taken up seriously in our universities. Professor Huxley said:

> The scholars of the medieval universities seem to have studied grammar, logic, and rhetoric; arithmetic and geometry; astronomy, theology, and music. Thus their work, however imperfect and faulty, judged by modern lights, it may have been, brought them face to face with all the leading aspects of the many-sided mind of man. For these studies did really contain, at any rate in embryo, sometimes it may be in caricature, what we now call philosophy, mathematical and physical science, and art. *And I doubt if the curriculum of any modern university shows so clear and generous a comprehension of what is meant by culture, as this old Trivium and Quadrivium does.*

It would be entirely a mistake, however, to think that these great writers and teachers who influenced the medieval universities so deeply and whose works were the text-books of the universities for centuries after, only had the principles of physical and experimental science and did not practically apply them. As a matter of fact their works are full of observation. Once more, the presumption that they wrote only nonsense with regard to science comes from those who do not know their writings at all, while great scientists who have taken the pains to study their works are enthusiastic in praise. Humboldt, for instance, says of Albertus Magnus, after reading some of his works with care:

> Albertus Magnus is equally active and influential in promoting the study of natural

> science and of the Aristotelian philosophy. His works contain some exceedingly acute remarks on the organic structure and physiology of plants. One of his works bearing the title of "Liber Cosmographicus De Natura Locorum" is a species of physical geography. I have found in it considerations on the dependence of temperature concurrently on latitude and elevation and on the effect of different angles of the sun's rays in heating the ground which have excited my surprise.

> It is with regard to physical geography of course that Humboldt is himself a distinguished authority.

Humboldt's expression that he found some exceedingly acute remarks on the organic structure and physiology of plants in Albert the Great's writings will prove a great surprise to many people. Meyer, the German historian of botany, however, has re-echoed Humboldt's praise with emphasis. The extraordinary erudition and originality of Albert's treatise on plants drew from Meyer the comment:

> No botanist who lived before Albert can be compared with him unless Theophrastus, with whom he was not acquainted; and after him none has painted nature in such living colors or studied it so profoundly until the time of Conrad Gessner and Cæsalpino.

These men, it may be remarked, come three centuries after Albert's time. A ready idea of Albert's contributions to physical science can be obtained from his life by Sighart, which has been translated into English by Dixon and was published in London in 1870. Pagel, in Puschmann's "History of Medicine," already referred to, gives a list of the books written by Albert on scientific matters with some comments which are eminently suggestive, and furnish solid basis for the remark that I have made, that men's minds were occupied with nearly the same problems in science in the thirteenth century as we are now, while the conclusions they came to were not very different from ours, though reached so long before us. This catalogue of Albertus Magnus' works shows very well his own interest and that of his generation in physical science of all kinds. There were eight treatises on Aristotle's physics and on the underlying principles of natural philosophy and of energy and of movement; four treatises concerning the heavens and the earth, one on physical geography which also contains, according to Pagel, numerous suggestions on ethnography and physiology. There are two treatises on generation and corruption, six books on meteors, five books on minerals, three books on the soul, two books on the intellect, a treatise on nutritives, and then a treatise on the senses and another on the memory and on the imagination. All the phases of the biological sciences were especially favorite subjects of his study. There is a treatise on the motion of animals, a treatise in six books on vegetables and plants, a treatise on breathing things, a treatise on sleep and waking, a treatise on youth and old age, and a treatise on life and death. His treatise on minerals contains, according to Pagel, a description of ninety-five different kinds of precious stones. Albert's volumes on plants were reproduced with Meyer, the German botanist, as editor (Berlin, 1867). All of Albert's books are available in modern editions.

Pagel says of Albertus that

> His profound scholarship, his boundless industry, the almost incontrollable impulse of his mind after universality of knowledge, the many-sidedness of his literary productivity, and finally the almost universal recognition which he received from his contemporaries and succeeding generations, stamp him as one of the most imposing characters and one of the most wonderful phenomena of the Middle Ages.

In another passage Pagel has said:

> While Albert was a Churchman and an ardent devotee of Aristotle, in matters of natural phenomena he was relatively unprejudiced and presented an open mind. He thought that he must follow Hippocrates and Galen, rather than Aristotle and Augustine, in medicine and in the natural sciences. We must concede it a special subject of praise for Albert that he distinguished very strictly between natural and supernatural phenomena. The former he considered as entirely the object of the investigation of nature. The latter he handed over to the realm of metaphysics.

Roger Bacon is, however, the one of these three great teachers who shows us how thoroughly practical was the scientific knowledge of the universities and how much it led to important useful discoveries in applied science and to anticipations of what is most novel even in our present-day sciences. Some of these indeed are so startling, that only that we know them not by tradition but from his works, where they may be readily found without any doubt of their authenticity, we should be sure to think that they must be the result of later commentators' ideas. Bacon was very much interested in astronomy, and not only suggested the correction of the calendar, but also a method by which it could be kept from wandering away from the actual date thereafter. He discovered many of the properties of lenses and is said to have invented spectacles and announced very emphatically that light did not travel instantaneously but moved with a definite velocity. He is sometimes said to have invented gunpowder, but of course he did not, though he studied this substance in various forms very carefully and drew a number of conclusions in his observations. He was sure that some time or other man would learn to control the energies exhibited by explosives and that then he would be able to accomplish many things that seemed quite impossible under present conditions.

He said, for instance:

> Art can construct instruments of navigation, such that the largest vessels governed by a single man will traverse rivers and seas more rapidly than if they were filled with oarsmen.

> One may also make carriages which without the aid of any animal will run with remarkable swiftness.

In these days when the automobile is with us and when the principal source of energy for motor purposes is derived from explosives of various kinds, this expression of Roger Bacon represents a prophecy marvellously surprising in its fulfilment. It is no wonder that the book whence it comes bears the title "De Secretis Artis et Naturæ." Roger Bacon even went to the extent, however, of declaring that man would some time be able to fly. He was even sure that with sufficient pains he could himself construct a flying machine. He did not expect to use explosives for his motor power, however, but thought that a windlass properly arranged, worked by hand, might enable a man to make sufficient movement to carry himself aloft or at least to support himself in the air, if there were enough surface to enable him to use his lifting power to advantage. He was in intimate relations by letter with many other distinguished inventors and investigators besides Peregrinus and was a source of incentive and encouragement to them all.

The more one knows of Aquinas the more surprise there is at his anticipation of many modern scientific ideas. At the conclusion of a course on cosmology delivered at the University of Paris he said that "nothing at all would ever be reduced to nothingness" (*nihil omnino in nihilum redigetur*). He was teaching the doctrine that man could not destroy matter and God would not annihilate it. In other words, he was teaching the indestructibility of matter even more emphatically than we do. He saw the many changes that take place in material substances around us, but he taught that these were only changes of form and not substantial changes and that the same amount of matter always remained in the world. At the same time he was teaching that the forms in matter by which he meant the combinations of energies which distinguish the various kinds of matter are not destroyed. In other words, he was anticipating not vaguely, but very clearly and definitely, the conservation of energy. His teaching with regard to the composition of matter was very like that now held by physicists. He declared that matter was composed of two principles, prime matter and form. By *forma* he meant the dynamic element in matter, while by *materia prima* he meant the underlying substratum of material, the same in every substance, but differentiated by the dynamics of matter.

It used to be the custom to make fun of these medieval scientists for believing in the transmutation of metals. It may be said that all three of these greatest teachers did not hold the doctrine of the transmutation of metals in the exaggerated way in which it appealed to many of their contemporaries. The theory of matter and form, however, gave a philosophical basis for the idea that one kind of matter might be changed into another. We no longer think that notion absurd. Sir William Ramsay has actually succeeded in changing one element into another and radium and helium are seen changing into each other, until now we are quite ready to think of transmutation placidly. The Philosopher's Stone used to seem a great absurdity until our recent experience with radium, which is to some extent at least the philosopher's stone, since it brings about the change of certain supposed elements into others. A distinguished American chemist said not long ago that he would like to extract all the silver from a large body of lead ore in which it occurs so commonly, and then come back after twenty years and look for further traces of silver, for he felt sure that they would be found and that lead ore is probably always producing silver in small quantities and copper ore is producing gold.

Most people will be inclined to ask where the fruits of this undergraduate teaching of science are to be found. They are inclined to presume that science was a closed book to the men and women of that time. It is not hard, however, to point the effect of the scientific training in the writings of the times. Dante is a typical university man of the period. He was at several Italian universities, was at Paris and perhaps at Oxford. His writings are full of science. Professor Kühns, of Wesleyan, in his book "The Treatment of Nature in Dante," has pointed out how much Dante knows of science and of nature. Few of the poets not only of his own but of any time have known more. There are only one or two writers of poetry in our time who go with so much confidence to nature and the scientific interpretation of her for figures for their poetry. The astronomy, the botany, the zoölogy of Albertus Magnus and Thomas Aquinas, Dante knew very well and used confidently for figurative purposes. Anyone who is inclined to think nature study a new idea in the world forgets, or has never known, his Dante. The birds and the bees, the flowers, the leaves, the varied aspects of clouds and sea, the phenomena of phosphorescence, the intimate habits of bird and beast and the ways of the plants, as well as all the appearances of the heavens, Dante knew very well and in a detail that is quite surprising when we recall how little nature study is supposed to have attracted the men of his time. Only that his readers appreciated it all, Dante would surely not have used his scientific erudition so constantly.

So much for the undergraduate department of the universities of the Middle Ages, and the view is absolutely fair, for these were the men to whom the students flocked by thousands. They were teaching science, not literature. They were discussing physics as well as metaphysics, psychology in its phenomena as well as philosophy, observation and experiment as well as logic, the ethical sciences, economics, practically all the scientific ideas that were needed in their generation—and that generation saw the rise of the universities, the finishing of the cathedrals, the building of magnificent town halls and castles and beautiful municipal buildings of many kinds, including hospitals, the development of the Hansa League in commerce, and of wonderful manufacturers of all the textiles, the arts and crafts, as well as the most beautiful book-making and art and literature. We could be quite sure that the men who solved all the other problems so well could not have been absurd only in their treatment of science. Anyone who reads their books will be quite sure of that.

While most people might be ready, then, to confess that possibly Huxley was not mistaken with regard to the undergraduate department of the universities, most of them would feel sure that at least the graduate departments were sadly deficient in accomplishment. Once more this is entirely an assumption. The facts are all against any such idea.

There were three graduate departments in most of the universities—theology, law, and medicine. While physical scientists are usually not cognizant of it apparently, theology is a science, a department of knowledge developed scientifically, and most of these medieval universities did more for its scientific development than the schools of any other period. Quite as much may be said for philosophy, for there are many who hesitate to attribute any scientific quality to modern developments in the matter. As for law, this is the great period of the foundation of scientific law development; the English common law was formulated by Bracton, the deep foundations of basic French and Spanish law were laid, and canon law acquired a definite scientific character which it was always to retain. All this was accomplished almost entirely by the professors in the law departments of the universities.

It was in medicine, however, where most people would be quite sure without any more ado that nothjing worth while talking about was being done, that the great triumphs of graduate teaching at the medieval universities were secured. Here more than anywhere else is there room for supreme surprise at the quite unheard-of anticipations of our modern medicine and, stranger still, as it may seem, of our modern surgery.

The law regulating the practice of medicine in the Two Sicilies about the middle of the thirteenth century shows us the high standard of medical education. Students were required to have three years of preliminary study at the university, four years in the medical department, and then practise for a year with a physician before they were allowed to practise for themselves. If they wanted to practise surgery, an extra year in the study of anatomy was required. I published the text of this law, which was issued by the Emperor Frederick II about 1241, in the *Journal of the American Medical Association* three years ago. It also regulated the practice of pharmacy. Drugs were manufactured under the inspection of the government and there was a heavy penalty for substitution, or for the sale of old inert drugs, or improperly prepared pharmaceutical materials. If the government inspector violated his obligations as to the oversight of drug preparations the penalty was death. Nor was this law of the Emperor Frederick an exception. We have the charters of a number of medical schools issued by the Popes during the next century, all of which require seven years or more of university study, four of them in the medical department, before the doctor's degree could be obtained. When new medical schools were founded they had to have professors from certain well-recognized schools on their staff at the beginning in order to assure proper standards of teaching, and all examinations were conducted under oath-bound secrecy and with the heaviest obligations on professors to be assured of the knowledge of students before allowing them to pass.

It might be easy to think, and many people are prone to do so, that in spite of the long years of study required there was really very little to study in medicine at that time. Those who think so should read Professor Clifford Allbutt's address on the "Historical Relations of Medicine and Surgery" delivered at the World's Fair at St. Louis in 1904. He has dwelt more on surgery than on medicine, but he makes it very clear that he considers that the thinking professors of medicine of the later Middle Ages were doing quite as serious work in their way as any that has been done since. They were carefully studying cases and writing case histories, they were teaching at the bedside, they were making valuable observations, and they were using the means at their command to the best advantage. Of course there are many absurdities in their therapeutics, but then we must not forget there have always been many absurdities in therapeutics and that we are not free from them in our day. Professor Richet, at the University of Paris, said not long ago: "The therapeutics of any generation is quite absurd to the second succeeding generation." We shall not blame the medieval generations for having accepted remedies that afterwards proved inert, for every generation has done that, even our own.

Their study of medicine was not without lasting accomplishment, however. They laid down the indications and the dosage for opium. They used iron with success, they tried out many of the bitter tonics among the herbal medicines, and they used laxatives and purgatives to good advantage. Down at Montpellier, Gilbert, the Englishman, suggested red light for smallpox because it shortened the fever, lessened the lesions, and made the disfigurement much less. Finsen was given the Nobel prize partly for rediscovery of this. They segregated erysipelas and so prevented its spread. They recognized the contagiousness of leprosy, and though it was probably as widespread as tuberculosis is at the present time, they succeeded not only in controlling but in eventually obliterating it throughout Europe.

It was in surgery, however, that the greatest triumphs of teaching of the medieval universities were secured. Most people are inclined to think that surgery developed only in our day. The great surgeons of the thirteenth and fourteenth centuries, however, anticipated most of our teaching. They investigated the causes of the failure of healing by first intention, recognized the danger of wounds of the neck, differentiated the venereal diseases, described rabies, and knew much of blood poisoning, and operated very skilfully. We have their text-books of surgery and they are a never-ending source of surprise. They operated on the brain, on the thorax, on the abdominal cavity, and did not hesitate to do most of the operations that modern surgeons do. They operated for hernia by the radical cure, though Mondeville suggested that more people were operated on for hernia for the benefit of the doctor's pocket than for the benefit of the patient. Guy de Chauliac declared that in wounds of the intestines patients would die unless the intestinal lacerations were sewed up, and he described the method of suture and invented a needle holder. We have many wonderful instruments from these early days preserved in pictures at least, that show us how much modern advance is merely re-invention.

They understood the principles of aseptic surgery very well. They declared that it was not necessary "that pus should be generated in wounds." Professor Clifford Allbutt says:

> They washed the wound with wine, scrupulously removing every foreign particle; then they brought the edges together, not allowing wine or anything else to remain

> within—dry adhesive surfaces were their desire. Nature, they said, produces the means of union in a viscous exudation, or natural balm, as it was afterwards called by Paracelsus, Paré, and Wurtz. In older wounds they did their best to obtain union by cleansing, desiccation, and refreshing of the edges. Upon the outer surface they laid only lint steeped in wine. Powders they regarded as too desiccating, for powder shuts in decomposing matters; wine after washing, purifying, and drying the raw surfaces evaporates.

Almost needless to say these are exactly the principles of aseptic surgery. The wine was the best antiseptic that they could use and we still use alcohol in certain cases. It would seem to many quite impossible that such operations as are described could have been done without anæsthetics, but they were not done without anæsthetics. There were two or three different forms of anæsthesia used during the thirteenth and fourteenth centuries. One method employed by Ugo da Lucca consisted of the use of an inhalant. We do not know what the material employed was. There are definite records, however, of its rather frequent employment.

What a different picture of science at the medieval universities all this makes from what we have been accustomed to hear and read with regard to them. It is difficult to understand where the old false impressions came from. The picture of university work that recent historical research has given us shows us professors and students busy with science in every department, making magnificent advances, many of which were afterwards forgotten, or at least allowed to lapse into desuetude.

The positive assertions with regard to old-time ignorance were all made in the course of religious controversy. In English-speaking countries particularly it became a definite purpose to represent the old Church as very much opposed to education of all kinds and above all to scientific education. There is not a trace of that to be found anywhere, but there were many documents that were appealed to to confirm the protestant view. There was a Papal bull, for instance, said to forbid dissection. When read it proves to forbid the cutting up of bodies to carry them to a distance for burial, an abuse which caused the spread of disease, and was properly prohibited. The Church prohibition was international and therefore effective. At the time the bull was issued there were twenty medical schools doing dissection in Italy and they continued to practise it quite undisturbed during succeeding centuries. The Papal physicians were among the greatest dissectors. Dissections were done at Rome and the cardinals attended them. Bologna at the height of its fame was in the Papal States. All this has been ignored and the supposed bull against anatomy emphasized as representing the keynote of medical and surgical history. Then there was a Papal decree forbidding the making of gold and silver. This was said to forbid chemistry or alchemy and so prevent scientific progress. The history of the medical schools of the time shows that it did no such thing. The great alchemists of the time doing really scientific work were all clergymen, many of them very prominent ecclesiastics.

Just in the same way there were said to be decrees of the Church councils forbidding the practice of surgery. President White says in his "Warfare of Science with Theology in Christendom," that, as a consequence of these, surgery was in dishonor until the Emperor Wenceslaus, at the beginning of the fifteenth century, ordered that it should be restored to estimation. As a matter of fact, during the two centuries immediately preceding the first years of the fifteenth century, surgery developed very wonderfully, and we have probably the most successful period in all the history of surgery except possibly our own. The decrees forbade monks to practise surgery because it led to certain abuses.Those who found these decrees and wanted to believe that they prevented all surgical development simply quoted them and assumed there was no surgery. The history of surgery at this time is one of the most wonderful chapters in human progress.

The more we know of the Middle Ages the more do we realize how much they accomplished in every department of intellectual effort. Their development of the arts and crafts has never been equalled in the modern time. They made very great literature, marvellous architecture, sculpture that rivals the Greeks', painting that is still the model for our artists, surpassing illuminations; everything that they touched became so beautiful as to be a model for all the after time. They accomplished as much in education as they did in all the other arts, their universities had more students than any that have existed down to our own time, and they were enthusiastic students and their professors were ardent teachers, writers, observers, investigators. While we have been accustomed to think of them as neglecting science, their minds were occupied entirely with science. They succeeded in anticipating much more of our modern thought, and even scientific progress, than we have had any idea until comparatively recent years. The work of the later Middle Ages in mathematics is particularly strong, and was the incentive for many succeeding generations. Roger Bacon insisted that, without mathematics, there was no possibility of real advance in physical science. They had the right ideas in every way. While they were occupied more with the philosophical and ethical sciences than we are, these were never pursued to the neglect of the physical sciences in the strictest sense of that term.

Is it not time that we should drop the foolish notions that are very commonly held because we know nothing about the Middle Ages—and, therefore, the more easily assume great knowledge—and get back to appreciate the really marvellous details of educational and scientific development which are so interesting and of so much significance at this time?

APPENDIX III

MEDIEVAL POPULARIZATION OF SCIENCE

The idea of collecting general information from many sources, of bringing it together into an easily available form, so as to save others labor, of writing it out in compendious fashion, so that it could readily pass from hand to hand, is likely to be considered typically modern. As a matter of fact, the Middle Ages furnish us with many examples of the popularization of science, of the writing of compendia of various kinds, of the gathering of information to save others the trouble, and, above all, of the making of what, in the modern time, we would call encyclopedias. Handbooks of various kinds were issued, manuals for students and specialists, and many men of broad scholarship in their time devoted themselves to the task of making the acquisition of knowledge easy for others. This was true not only for history and philosophy and literature, but also for science. It is not hard to find in each century of the Middle Ages some distinguished writer who devoted himself to this purpose, and for the sake of the light that it throws on these scholars, and the desire for information that must have existed very commonly since they were tempted to do the work, it seems worth while to mention here their names, and those of the books they wrote, with something of their significance, though the space will not permit us to give here much more than a brief *catalogue raisonné* of such works.

Very probably the first who should be mentioned in the list is Boëthius, who flourished in the early part of the sixth century. He owed much of his education to his adoptive father, afterwards his father-in-law, Symmachus, who, with Festus, represented scholarship at the court of the Gothic King, Theodoric of Verona. These three – Festus, Symmachus, and Boëthius – brought such a reputation for knowledge to the court that they are responsible for many of the wonderful legends of Dietrich of Bern, as Theodoric came to be called in the poems of the medieval German poets. The three distinguished and devoted scholars did much to save Greek culture at a time when its extinction was threatened, and Boëthius particularly left a series of writings that are truly encyclopedic in character. There are five books on music, two on arithmetic, one on geometry, translations of Aristotle's treatises on logic, with commentaries; of Porphyry's "Isagoge," with commentaries, and a commentary on Cicero's "Topica." Besides, he wrote several treatises in logic and rhetoric himself, one on the use of the syllogism, and one on topics, and in addition a series of theological works. His great "Consolations of Philosophy" was probably the most read book in the early Middle Ages. It was translated into Anglo-Saxon by King Alfred, into old German by Notker Teutonicus, the

German monk of St. Gall, and its influence may be traced in Beowulf, in Chaucer, in High German poetry, in Anglo-Norman and Provençal popular poetry, and also in early Italian verse. Above all, the "Divine Comedy" has many references to it, while the "Convito" would seem to show that it was probably the book that most influenced Dante. Though it is impossible to confirm by documentary evidence the generally accepted idea that Boëthius died a martyr for Christianity, the tradition can be traced so far back, and it has been so generally accepted that this seems surely to have been the case. The fact is interesting, as showing the attitude of scholars towards the Church and of the Church towards scholarship thus early.

The next great name in the tradition should probably be that of Cassiodorus, the Roman writer and statesman, prime minister of Theodoric, who, after a busy political life, retired to his estate at Vivarium, and, in imitation of St. Benedict, who had recently established a monastery at Monte Cassino, founded a monastery there. He is said to have lived to the age of ninety-three. His retirement favored this long life, for, after the death of Theodoric, troublous times came, and civil war, and only his monastic privileges saved him from the storm and stress of the times. He had been interested in literature and the collection of information of many kinds before his retirement, and it is not unlikely that his recognition of the fact that the monastic life offered opportunities for the pursuit of this, under favorable circumstances, led him to take it up.

While still a statesman he wrote a series of works relating to history and politics and public affairs generally. These consisted mainly of chronicles and panegyrics, and twelve books of miscellanies called Variæ. After his retirement to the monastery, a period of ardent devotion to writing begins, and a great number of books were issued. He evidently gathered round him a number of men whom he inspired with his spirit, or, perhaps, selected, because he found that, while they had a taste for a quiet, peaceful spiritual life, they were also devoted to the accumulation and diffusion of knowledge. A series of commentaries on portions of the Scriptures was written, the Jewish antiquities of Josephus translated, and the ecclesiastical histories of Theodoric, Sozomen, and Socrates made available in Latin. Cassiodorus himself is said to have made a compendium of these, called the "Historia Tripartita," which was much used as a manual of history during succeeding centuries. Then there were treatises on grammar, on orthography, and a series of works on mathematics. In all of his writings Cassiodorus shows a special fondness for the symbolism of numbers.

There is a well-grounded tradition that he insisted on the study of the Greek classics of medical literature, especially Hippocrates and Galen, and awakened the interest of the monks in the necessity for making copies of these fathers of medicine. The tradition that he established at Vivarium is also found to have existed at Monte Cassino among the Benedictines, and, doubtless, to this is to be attributed the foundation of the medical school of Salerno, where Benedictine influence was so strong. It is probable, therefore, that to Cassiodorus must be attributed the preservation in as perfect a state as we have them of the old Greek medical writers.

His main idea was, of course, the study of Scriptures, but with just as many helps as possible. He thought that commentators, and historians, not alone Christian, but also Hebrew and Pagan, should be studied to illustrate it, and then the commentaries of the Latin fathers, so that a thoroughly rounded knowledge of it should be obtained. He thus began an "Encyclopedia Biblica," and set a host of workers at its accomplishment.

Every country in Europe shared this movement for the diffusion of information during the early Middle Ages, and the works of men from each of these countries in succeeding centuries has come down to us, preserved in spite of all the vicissitudes to which they were so liable during the centuries before the invention of printing and the easy multiplication of books. To many people it will seem surprising to learn that the next evidence of deep broad interest in knowledge is to be found in the next century in the distant west of Europe, in the Spanish Peninsula. It is a long step from the semi-barbaric splendor of the Gothic court at Verona, to the bishop's palace in Seville in Andalusia. The two cities are separated by what is no inconsiderable distance in our day. In the seventh century they must have seemed almost at the other end of the world from each other. Those who recall what we have insisted on in several portions of the body of this work with regard to the high place Spanish genius won for itself in the Roman Empire, and how much of culture among the Spaniards of that time the occurrence of so many important writers of that nationality must imply, will not be surprised at the distinguished work of a great Christian Spanish writer of the seventh century.

Indeed, it would be only what might be expected for evidences of early awakening of the broadest culture to be found in Spain. The important name in the popularization of science in the seventh century is St. Isidore of Seville. He made a compendium of all the scattered scientific traditions and information of his time with regard to natural phenomena in a sort of encyclopedia of science. This consisted of twenty books—chapters we would call them now—treating almost *de omni re scibili et quibusdam aliis* (everything knowable and a few other things besides). It is possible that the work may have been written by a number of collaborators under the patronage of the bishop, though there is no sure indication of this to be found either in the volume itself or even contemporary history. All the ordinary scientific subjects are treated. Astronomy, geography, mineralogy, botany, and even man and the animals have each a special chapter. Pouchet, in his "History of the Natural Sciences During the Middle Ages," calls attention to the fact that, in grouping the animals for collective treatment in the different chapters, sometimes the most heterogeneous creatures are brought under a common heading. Among the fishes, for instance, are classed all living things that are found in water. The whale and the dolphin, as well as sponges, and oysters, and crocodiles, and sea serpents, and lobsters, and hippopotamuses, all find a place together, because of the common watery habitation. The early Spanish Churchman would seem to have had an enthusiastic zeal for complete classification that would surely have made him a strenuous modern zoölogist.

The next link in the tradition of encyclopedic work is the Venerable Bede, whose character was more fully honored by the decree on November 13, 1899, by Pope Leo XIII declaring him a Doctor of the Church. Bede was the fruit of that ardent scholarship which had risen in England as a consequence of the introduction of Christianity. It had been fostered by the coming of scholar saints from Ireland, but was, unfortunately, disturbed by the incursions of the Danes. While Bede is known for his greatest work, the "Ecclesiastical History of the English People," which gives an account of Christianity in England from its beginning until his own day, he wrote many other works. His history is the foundation of all our knowledge of early British history, secular as well as religious, and has been praised by historical writers of all ages, who turned to it for help with confidence. He wrote a number of other historical works. Besides, he wrote books on grammar, orthography, the metrical art, on rhetoric, on the nature of things, the seasons, and on the calculation of the seasons. These latter books are distinctly scientific. His contributions to Gregorian Music are now of great value.

After this, Alcuin and the monks, summoned by Charlemagne, take up the tradition of gathering and diffusing information, and the great monasteries of Tours, Fulda, and St. Gall carry it on. Besides these, in the ninth century Monte Cassino comes into prominence as an institution where much was done of what we would now call encyclopedic work. After his retirement from Salerno Constantine Africanus made his translations and commentaries on Arabian medicine, constituting what was really a medical encyclopedia of information not readily available at that time.

After this, of course, the tradition is taken up by the universities, and it is only when, with the thirteenth century, there came the complete development of the university spirit, that encyclopedias reached their modern expression. Three great encyclopedists, Vincent of Beauvais, Thomas of Cantimprato, and Bartholomæus Anglicus, are the most famous. Vincent consulted all the authors sacred and profane that he could lay hold on, and the number was, indeed, prodigious. I have given some account of him in "The Thirteenth Greatest of Centuries" (Catholic Summer School Press, New York, third edition, 1910).

It would be very easy to conclude that these encyclopedias, written by clergymen for the general information of the educated people of the times, contain very little that is scientifically valuable, and probably nothing of serious medical significance. Any such thought is, however, due entirely to unfamiliarity with the contents of these works. They undoubtedly contain absurdities, they are often full of misinformation, they repeat stories on dubious authority, and sometimes on hearsay, but usually the source of their information is stated, and especially where it is dubious, as if they did not care to state marvels without due support. Books of popular information, however, have always had many queer things,—queer, that is, to subsequent generations,—and it is rather amusing to pick up an encyclopedia of a century ago, much less a millennium ago, and see how many absurd things were accepted as true. The first edition of the "Encyclopedia Britannica," issued one hundred and fifty years ago, furnishes an easily available source of the absurdities our more recent forefathers accepted. The men of the Middle Ages, however, were much better observers as a rule, and used much more critical judgment, according to their lights, than we have given them credit for. Often the information that they have to convey is not only valuable, but well digested, thoroughly practical, and sometimes a marvellous anticipation of some of our most modern thoughts. There is one of these encyclopedias which, because it was written in my favorite thirteenth century, I have read with some care. It is simply a development of the work of preceding clerical encyclopedists, and often refers to them. Because it contains some typical examples of the better sorts of information in these works, I have thought it worth while to quote two passages from it. The author is Bartholomæus Anglicus, and the quaint English in which it is couched is quoted from "Medical Lore" (London, 1893). The book is all the more interesting because in a dear old English version, issued about 1540, the spellings of which are among the great curiosities of English orthography, it was often read and consulted by Shakespeare, who evidently quotes from it frequently, for not a little of the quaint scientific lore that he uses for his figures can be traced to expressions used in this book.

The first of the paragraphs that deserves to be quoted, discusses madness, or, as we would call it, lunacy, and sums up the causes, the symptoms, and the treatment quite as well as that has ever been done in the same amount of space:

> Madness cometh sometime of passions of the soul, as of business and of great thoughts, of sorrow and of too great study, and of dread: sometime of the biting of a wood hound, or some other venomous beast; sometime of melancholy meats, and sometime

> of drink of strong wine. And as the causes be diverse, the tokens and signs be diverse. For some cry and leap and hurt and wound themselves and other men, and darken and hide themselves in privy and secret places. The medicine of them is, that they be bound, that they hurt not themselves and other men. And namely, such shall be refreshed, and comforted, and withdrawn from cause and matter of dread and busy thoughts. And they must be gladded with instruments of music, and some deal be occupied.'

The second discusses in almost as thorough a way the result of the bite of a mad dog. The old English word for mad, wood, is constantly used. The causes, the symptoms, and course of the disease, and its possible prevention by early treatment, are all discussed. The old tradition was already in existence that sufferers from rabies or hydrophobia, as it is called, dreaded water, when it is really only because the spasm consequent upon the thought even of swallowing is painful that they turn from it. That tradition has continued to be very commonly accepted even by physicians down to our own day, so that Bartholomew, the Englishman, in the thirteenth century, will not be blamed much for setting it forth for popular information in his time some seven centuries ago. The idea that free bleeding would bring about the removal of the virus is interesting, because we have in recent years insisted in the case of the very similar disease, tetanus, on allowing or deliberately causing wounds in which the tetanus microbe may have gained an entrance, to bleed freely.

> The biting of a wood hound is deadly and venomous. And such venom is perilous. For it

is long hidden and unknown, and increaseth and multiplieth itself, and is sometimes unknown to the year's end, and then the same day and hour of the biting, it cometh to the head, and breedeth frenzy. They that are bitten of a wood hound have in their sleep dreadful sights, and are fearful, astonied, and wroth without cause. And they dread to be seen of other men, and bark as hounds, and they dread water most of all things, and are afeared thereof full sore and squeamous also. Against the biting of a wood hound wise men and ready use to make the wounds bleed with fire or with iron, that the venom may come out with the blood, that cometh out of the wound.

FOOTNOTES

[1]"Medicinisches aus der Aeltesten Kirchen Geschichte." Leipzig, 1892.

[2]Foulis, London and Edinburgh, 1910.

[3]My attention was called to the interesting story of the Jewish physicians of the Middle Ages and their scientific accomplishment while writing the article on Joseph Hyrtl for the Catholic Encyclopedia. His "Das Arabische und Hebräische in der Anatomie" (Wien, 1879) has some interestingly suggestive material on these important chapters of the history of medicine. (I owe my opportunity to consult it to the courtesy of the Surgeon-General's library.) Biographic material has been obtained from Carmoly's "History of the Jewish Physicians," translated by Dr. Dunbar for the Maryland Medical and Surgical Journal, some extra copies of which were printed by John Murphy and Co., Baltimore, about the middle of the nineteenth century. Baas and Haeser's Histories of

Medicine and Puschmann and Pagel's "Handbook" provided additional material, and I have found Landau's "Geschichte der Jüdischen Aerzte" (Berlin, 1895) of great service.

[4]Of course there are many absurd things recommended in the Talmud. We cannot remind ourselves too often, however, that there have been absurd things at all times in medicine, and especially in therapeutics. It is curious how often some of these absurdities have repeated themselves. We are liable to think it very queer that men should have presumed, or somehow jumped to the conclusion, that portions of animals might possess wonderful virtue for the healing of diseases of the corresponding special parts of man. We ourselves, however, within a little more than a decade, had a phase of opotherapy—how much less absurd it seems under that high-sounding Greek term—that was apparently very learned in its scientific aspects yet quite as absurd as many phases of old-time therapy, as we look at it. We administered cardin for heart disease and nephrin for kidney trouble, cerebrin for insanity (save the mark!), and even prostate tissue for prostatism—and with reported good results! How many of us realize now that in this we were only repeating the absurdities, so often made fun of in old medicine, with regard to animal tissue and excrement therapeutics? The Talmud has many conclusions with regard to the symptoms of patients drawn from dreams; as, for instance, it is said to be a certain sign of sanguineous plethora when one dreams of the comb of a cock. One phase of our psycho-analysis in the modern time, however, has taken us back to an interpretation of dreams different of course from this, yet analogous enough to be quite striking.

[5]"Maimonides," by David Yellin and Israel Abrahams, Philadelphia, 1903.

[6]"Das Arabische und Hebräische in der Anatomie," Dr. Joseph Hyrtl, Wien, 1879.

[7]"Anat. Antiq. Rariores," Vienna, 1835.

[8]It seems hard to understand how so useful an auxiliary to the surgeon as the ligature,—it seems indispensable to us,—could possibly be allowed to go out of use and even be forgotten. It will not be difficult, however, for anyone who recalls the conditions that obtained in old-time surgery. The ligature is a most satisfying immediate resource in stopping bleeding from an artery, but a septic ligature inevitably causes suppuration and almost inevitably leads to secondary hemorrhage. In the old days of septic surgery secondary hemorrhage was the surgeon's greatest and most dreaded bane. Some time from the fifth to the ninth day a septic ligature came away under conditions such that inflammatory disturbance had prevented sealing of the vessel. If the vessel was large, then the hemorrhage was fast and furious and the patient died in a few minutes. After a surgeon had had a few deaths of this kind he dreaded the ligature. He abandoned its use and took kindly to such methods as the actual cautery, red-hot knives for amputations, and the like, that would sear the surfaces of tissues and the blood-vessels, and not give rise to secondary hemorrhage. A little later, however, someone not familiar with secondary risks would reinvent the ligature. If he were cleanly in his methods and, above all, if he were doing his work in a new hospital, the ligature worked very well for a while. If not, it soon fell into innocuous desuetude again.

[9]Puschmann: "Handbuch der Geschichte der Medizin," Vol. I, page 652.

[10]The first dentist who filled teeth with amalgam in New York, some eighty years ago, had to flee for his life, because of a hue and cry set up that he was poisoning his patients with mercury.

[11]"Storia de la Scuola di Salerno."

[12]It is probably interesting to note that the word universitas as used here has no reference to our word university, but refers to the

whole world of students as it were. In the Middle Ages universities were called studia generalia, general studies—that is, places where everything could be studied and where everyone from any part of the world could study. Our use of the word university in the special modern sense of the term comes from the formal mode of address to the faculty of a university when Popes or rulers sent them authoritative documents. Such documents began with the expression Universitas vestra, all of you (in the old-time English, as preserved in the Irish expression, "the whole of ye"), referring to all the members of the faculty. The transfer to our term and signification university was not difficult.

[13]Physicians wore a particular garb consisting of a cloak and often a mask, supposed to protect them from infections at this time, so that it was not difficult to make a characteristic picture as a sign for a pharmacy. These symbolic signs were much commoner and very necessary when people generally were not able to read. It is from that period that we have the mortar and pestle as also the colored lights in the windows of the drug stores, and the many-colored barber-pole. Also the big boot, key, watch, hat, bonnet, and the like, the last symbolic sign invention apparently being the wooden Indian for the tobacco store.

[14]The Medical Library and Historical Journal, Brooklyn, December, 1906.

[15]Taddeo, who was born in 1215, according to our usually accepted traditions in the matter, would have been seventy-five years of age when Mondino as a youth of scarcely more than fifteen went to the University. It might seem that so old a man would have very little influence over the young man. Taddeo, however, had, as we have said, a very strenuous old age. Everything in life had come to him late. He was well past thirty before he began to study philosophy and medicine, having been a seller of candles from necessity because of poverty in his younger years. His great success

in practice came when he was past forty. He first began to teach when he was forty-five, and he was nearly fifty-five before he began to write. According to tradition he married when he was nearly eighty—whether for the first or second time is not said—and while this might be considered, and would in some cases be, an indication of weakness of character (it would probably depend on whether he married or was married), it seems in his case to have indicated a vigor of body and character which shows very clearly how great was the possibility of his influence as a teacher having been maintained even up to this late time of life, and thus influencing a pupil who is to represent the most potent influence at the beginning of the next century.

[16]Medical Library and Historical Journal, 1906.

[17]Pilcher (loc. cit.) tells of her tomb. I venture to change his translation of the inscription in certain unimportant particulars. He says:

"We know the very place where she was buried in front of the Madonna delle Lettre in the Church of San Pietro e Marcellino of the Hospital of Santa Maria de Mareto, where her associate, Agenio, mourning and inconsolable, placed a tablet with this inscription:

D . O . M .
Vrceo . Contenti
Alexandrae . Galinae . Pvellae . Persicetanae
Penicillo . Egregiae . Ad . Anatomen . Exhibendam
Et . Insignissimi . Medici . Mundini . Lucii
Paucis . Comparandae . Discipulae . Cineres
Carnis . Hic . Expectant . Resurrectionem
Vixit . Ann . XIX . Obiit . Studio . Absunta
Die XXVI Martii . A . S . MCCCXXVI
Otto . Agenius . Lustrulanus . Ob . Eam . Demptam

Sui . Potiori . Parte . Spoliatus . Sodali . Eximiae
Ac . De . Se . Optime . Meritae . Inconsolabilis . M . P .

This inscription may be translated as follows:

In this urn enclosed
The ashes of the body of
Alexandra Giliani, a maiden of Periceto;
Skilful with her brush in anatomical demonstrations
And a disciple equalled by few,
Of the most noted physician, Mundinus of Luzzi,
Await the resurrection.
She lived 19 years: she died consumed by her labors
March 26, in the year of grace 1326.
Otto Agenius Lustrulanus, by her taking away
Deprived of his better part, his excellent companion,
Deserving of the best,
Has erected this tablet."

[18]This is so striking that I quote their actual words from Gurlt, p. 704: "Multoties fit percussio in anteriori parte cranei et craneum in parte frangitur contraria."

[19]"Historical Relations of Medicine and Surgery Down to the Sixteenth Century," London, 1904.

[20]Of course, for any extended knowledge of Mondeville, a modern reader must turn to Nicaise's translation of his "Chirurgia," which, with an introduction and a biography, was published at Paris in 1893. Nicaise's publication of this and of Guy de Chauliac's treatise has worked a revolution in medical history and, above all, has made these old authors available for those who hesitate to take up a work written entirely in Latin.

[21]In the very first book containing some account of human anatomy, a German volume by Conradus Mengenberger, called

"Puch der Natur," the date of printing of which is about 1478,—that is, less than ten years after the printing of the very first book, the "Biblia pauperum," which appeared in 1470,—there are, according to Haller in his "Bibliotheca Anatomica," a series of illustrations. This is the first illustrated medical work ever published.

[22]Fordham University Press, New York, 1908.

[23]Fordham University Press, New York, 1908.

[24]See picture of the hospital ward at Tonnerre, in "The Thirteenth Greatest of Centuries," 3rd edit., New York, 1911.

[25]"The Historical Relations of Medicine and Surgery," by T. Clifford Allbutt, M.A., M.D. London: Macmillan & Co., Ltd., 1905.

[26]The beginning of the manuscript copy in the "Bibliothèque Nationale" is extremely interesting as an example of the English of the period, and alongside of it it seems worth while to quote the closing sentence as Nicaise reproduces them:

"In godes name here bygyneth the inventarie of gadryng to gedre medecyne in the partye of cyrurgie compilede and fulfilled in the zere (yere?) of our Loord 1363 by Guide de Cauliaco cirurgene and doctor of physik in the fulclere studye of Mountpylerz.

"On page 191, verso.—Here endeth the cyrurgie of Maistre Guyd' de Cauliaco dottoure of phisik."

The University of Cambridge copy has the title in the colophon. It runs as follows: "Ye inventorye of Guydo de Caulhiaco Doctor of Phisyk and Cirurgien in Ye Universitie of Mount Pessulanee of Montpeleres." The fly-leaf contains the words, "Jesu Christ save ye soule of mich." It is rather interesting to note how much closer to modern English is this copy, made probably not much more than half a century later than the first one and, above all, how much more nearly the spelling has come. At this time, however, and, indeed, for more than a century later, spelling had no fixed rule, and a man might spell the same word quite differently even on the same page. The difference between doctor spelled thus in the early edition, and doctours in the later one, probably means nothing more than personal peculiarities of the original translator or copyist.

[27]In Nicaise this last word is written crapte. I have ventured to suggest crafte, since a misreading between the two letters would be so easy. In the same way I have suggested tentatively a changing of the z in the title of the Bibliothèque Nationale copy to y, making the word yere instead of zere.

[28]"A History of Dentistry from the Most Ancient Times Until the End of the Eighteenth Century," by Dr. Vincenzo Guerini, editor of the Italian Review L'Odonto-Stomatologia, Philadelphia and New York, Lea and Febriger, 1909.

[29]The first printed edition of Arculanus is that of Venice, 1542, bearing the Latin title, "Joannis Arculani Commentaria in Nonum Librum Rasis," etc.

[30]It is curious to trace how old are the traditions on which some of these old stories, that must now be rejected, are founded. I have come upon the story with regard to Basil Valentine and the antimony and the monks in an old French medical encyclopedia of biography, published in the seventeenth century, and at that time there was no doubt at all expressed as to its truth. How much older than this it may be I do not know, though it is probable that it comes from the sixteenth century, when the kakoëthes scribendi attacked many people because of the facility of printing, and when most of the good stories that have so worried the modern dry-as-dust historian in his researches for their correction became a part of the body of supposed historical tradition. It is probably French in origin because in that language antimoine is a tempting bait for that pseudo-philology which has so often led to false derivations.

[31]There is in the New York Academy of Medicine a thick 24mo volume in which three of the classics of older medicine are bound together. They are Kerckringius's "Commentary on the Triumphal Chariot of Antimony," published at Amsterdam, 1671; Steno's "Dissertation on the Anatomy of the Brain," published in Leyden in 1671, and Father Kircher's "Scrutinium Physico Contagiosae Luis quae dicitur Pestis" (Physico-medical Discussions of the Contagious Disease which is called Pest). This was published at Leipzig in 1659. Just how the three works came to be bound together is hard to say. Very probably they belonged to some old-time scholar, though there is nothing about the books to tell anything of the story. The fact that all three of the authors were ecclesiastics of the Catholic Church, Valentine a Monk, Steno a Bishop, and Kircher a Jesuit, would seem to be one common bond and perhaps a reason for the binding of these rather disparate treatises together. In that case it is probable that the book came from an old monastic library dispersed after the suppression of the order by some government. It seems not unlikely that the volume belonged at some time to an old Jesuit library, for they have suffered the most in that way. That these three classics of medicine should have been republished in handy volume editions within practically ten years shows an interest in medical literature that has not existed again until our own time, for during the eighteenth and early nineteenth centuries there was almost utter neglect of them.

[32]Paper read before the first meeting of the American Guild of St. Luke.

[33]Published by Putnams, New York, 1909.

[34]Dublin, 1882.

[35]The material for this chapter was gathered for a paper read before the Medical Improvement Society of Boston in the spring of 1911. In nearly its present form it was published in The Popular

Science Monthly for May, 1911, and thanks are returned to the editor of that magazine for permission to reprint it here. The additions that have been made refer particularly to the estimation of Aristotle in the Middle Ages.

[36]New York, Putnam, 1908.

[37]"De Cœlo et Mundo," 1, tr. iv., x.

INDEX

•F

LITERARY CRITIQUES

Dr. James J. Walsh's "Old-Time Maker's of Medicine" is an extensive study of the history of medicine which examines the life as well as efforts of first medical professionals and thinkers. The writer offers an extensive review of the development of medical thought as well as practice from ancient to Renaissance times in this publication. Here's a quick summary & analysis: Folk Cures as well as Early Medicine:

Religious views were oftentimes intertwined with medical procedures in the early days. The main healers were Shamans, priests and smart women.

Early practitioners utilized herbal cures, rituals, and chants for treatment of problems.

The pharmacology was established by using real medicinal plants and herbs.

Greek Medicine:

The Greeks changed the focus from spiritual to logical and observational.

Hippocrates: He was frequently credited with introducing the notion of diseases being natural events and not divine punishments. He advocated for clinical examination, prognosis and patient secrecy.

Doctors today still swear the Hippocratic Oath which highlights ethics in medicine.

Dioscorides is among the noteworthy writers who published extensively on the medicinal plants and properties.

Roman Medicine:

Romans integrated Greek medical knowledge, but additionally contributed with their knowledge in public health and sanitation.

Galen: His enormous works merged philosophy, anatomy and medicine. Despite several of his theories, particularly concerning humors, being later proved incorrect, his influence continued for centuries and was unmatched.

The surgical instruments as well as methods of Romans were likewise notable advancements.

Arabic Medicine:

The Islamic world acted as a model of learning throughout the European Dark Ages.

Avicenna (IBn Sina) and other medical giants authored "The Canon of Medicine," resulting in a 5 volume encyclopedia that became renowned throughout Europe for centuries.

Another significant writer was Al-Razi (Rahazes) who published extensively on illnesses like measles and smallpowder, stressing empirical observation.

Medieval Medicine:

European monasteries preserved old medical texts and turned into centers of healing, with monks doubling as doctors.

The School of Salerno in southern Italy had been a crucial institution integrating Greek, Roman, Arabic and Jewish medical knowledge. The initial phases of formal medical education began here too.

The emergence of apothecaries (early pharmacists) and barber - surgeon triggered a proliferation in medieval Europe.

Renaissance Medicine:

There had been a renewal of curiosity in human anatomy and a challenging of older doctrines during this era.

Andreas Vesalius :. The work "De humani corpori s fabrica" revolutionized anatomy and fixed a number of Galen's mistakes.

The printing press of the 15th century became a significant advancement in facilitating the widespread transmission of medical information.

Innovative discoveries concerning the circulatory system by William Harvey further shifted the understanding of the body.

LITERARY ANALYSIS

The Meaning of Observation: The value of attentive observation and documentation is stressed throughout the book. The focus on direct observation provided the groundwork for contemporary scientific inquiry, beginning from Hippocrates' clinical observations through Al-Razi's empiricist approach.

Cultural Exchange and its Impact: The interaction between diverse civilizations enriched medical knowledge. The Arabs translated and preserved Greek and Rome texts, which they later distributed to Europe.

Defying Established Laws: The Renaissance period stresses the significance of challenging established knowledge. Vesalius along with other figures that challenged Galenic teachings produced substantial backlash but perseverance led to progress.

Holistic Approach: The Greek and Arabic traditions of ancient practitioners were recognized for viewing health holistically, covering the mind, body as well as environment. The emphasis in contemporary medicine on lifestyle, mental health, along with preventive care is revitalizing this viewpoint.

The Department of Institutional Support: Institutions were integral to fostering and spreading medical knowledge, starting with monastic communities and continuing through universities. They not only provided information but also a collaborative place for debate and discussion.

Essentially, "Old-Time Makers of Medicine" underscores the journey of medical knowledge, marked by individual genius, cultural exchanges, challenges to established norms, and the undying human pursuit for understanding and healing.

"Old-Time Maker of Medicine: Historical Background"

"Old-Time Maker - of Medicine" covers a period from early civilizations to the Renaissance - a very long time span which witnessed empires rise and fall, religions spread and fantastic intellectual and medical developments.

Ancient Civilizations: The Egyptians, Sumerians as well as Indus Valley societies had basic medical methods as did other ancient cultures. They had been profoundly spiritually based, with diseases frequently connected with divine resentment or bad spirits. The surgical procedures, herbal cures and healing rituals are detailed in hieroglyphics and old scroll of this time.

Golden Age of Greece: Around the 5th as well as 4th centuries BCE, Greece underwent a rush of intellectual activity. Thinkers like Socrates, Aristotle, and Plato challenged the nature of existence, society, and expertise. The spirit of inquiry extended to medicine, where figures like Hippocrates stressed natural explanations for ailments.

Roman Empire: Throughout their peak, the Romans widened their reach into Europe, North Africa along with West Asia. They were also distinguished for their engineering abilities that impacted public health through aquiducts, sewers and baths. While they incorporated much of Greek medicine they also brought their very own practical approach, particularly in surgery.

Islamic Golden Age: The Islamic world flourished as the Roman Empire declined and Europe entered into the Dark Ages. The Middle East underwent a surge in scientific, literary and philosophical endeavors from the 8th to 13th centuries CE. Arab experts translated and preserved ancient Greek and Roman texts, making sure their survival.

The medieval Europe era: The early Middle Ages in Europe had been marked by feudalism, with society organized around castles and manors. The Church dominated all areas of life. Monasteries became libraries of learning, along with monks frequently acted as healers due to their access to ancient texts. University establishment in the 12th century had been a signal of rekindled interest in learning.

The Renaissance: The Renaissance is a social and intellectual revitalization which spans the 14th to 17th centuries. It started in Italy and sprang up throughout Europe. The rebirth of interest in ancient Greek and

Roman texts produced philosophical, scientific, and artistic accomplishments in large numbers. This required a change in medicine from dogmatic obedience to early authorities to direct observation as well as examination.

Medicine turned into a systematic discipline all through these times, transforming from mystical rituals to. This evolution was mostly because of the exchange of knowledge across cultures, the contribution of key people challenging established norms and institutional backing. The basis for the scientific revolution and modern medical science were laid in the Renaissance.

Understanding this historical context helps readers appreciate the myriad factors which shaped the development of medical thought as well as practice, as documented in "Old-Time Makers of Medicine".

CONTENT

www.ingramcontent.com/pod-product-compliance
Lightning Source LLC
LaVergne TN
LVHW011632200926
848484LV00010B/2536